Crouched, waving the knife, Melissa looked at John. "Don't come any closer." As she watched, an angry smile changed John's face into something horrible, and Melissa realized that this had gone much too far. "Calm down, baby," she said, straightening. "It's okay now. We can talk about this. . . ."

Slowly John walked toward her. "You gotta learn some respect for your husband."

"Don't, John baby," Melissa said, her voice now a whine.

"Yeah. Some respect."

Later, as she tried to tell the authorities exactly what happened next, she said that she didn't know. Exactly who moved first and how was a blank. She said she recalled nothing except John on the floor, blood seeping from his chest, the bloody knife still in her hand. . . .

By Joan E. Lloyd and Edwin B. Herman:

RESCUE ALERT
DIAL 911*
LIGHTS AND SIREN*
TRAUMA CENTER*
EMT: RACE FOR LIFE*

Published by Ivy Books

EMT:
Race for Life

Joan E. Lloyd
and Edwin B. Herman

IVY BOOKS • NEW YORK

An Ivy Book
Published by The Ballantine Publishing Group
Copyright © 1998 by Joan E. Lloyd and Edwin B. Herman

Grateful acknowledgment is made to JEMS, FIRE RESCUE and EMS Insider for permission to reprint a poem, *Song of the EMT*, by Thom Dick. Copyright © 1981 by Thom Dick, EMT-P.

http://www.randomhouse.com

Library of Congress Catalog Card Number: 98-96100

ISBN 0-8041-1545-1

Manufactured in the United States of America

First Edition: October 1998

10 9 8 7 6 5 4 3 2 1

Dedication

To Danny N., our dear friend, whom we miss so much.
May the bluefish be running wherever you are.
And to Danny C., whom we never got to know.
We tried so hard.

Chapter 1

Mindy Okamura loved staying home and being a full-time mother. After her son John's birth four years earlier, she had tried to continue working. "I want to feel like I'm contributing," she would say, but, when she became pregnant for the second time, her husband finally convinced her to quit her job and stay at home. And once Barbara arrived, Mindy wondered why she had ever considered trying to work.

Each evening she carefully planned activities that were both fun and educational for the children. She quickly found that she was putting as much energy into her family as she had into her job.

At four and two, the children had lively minds, which Mindy loved to feed. She read to them, colored numbers and letters, did science projects, and haunted the educational toy stores for new ideas. Both John and Babs had gymnastics lessons, church school on Sundays, and play dates with various other children.

One late spring morning Mindy had gotten out the plastic shoe box with the crayons and markers and the three of them were about to make pictures of birds. "Let's do this outside on the patio table," Mindy suggested, and the three, carrying paper, the marker box, and

Babs's booster chair, trooped out to the patio and set up their art project on the glass table. For fifteen minutes, longer than Babs's usual attention span, they used red markers for cardinals and blue ones for jays. While drawing, they listened to the early-morning bird music from the wooded area behind the house. "Listen," Mindy said. "We're coloring a robin and there's his song."

"Mama, down," Babs demanded.

"Okay, honey," Mindy said. "Just one more bit of color here on the bird's belly."

"Mama, down." Babs wiggled and, as she had just learned to do, unsnapped the restraining strap that held her in the booster chair.

No one was ever really sure exactly what happened during the next few seconds. Babs's chair tipped, the table umbrella shifted, and suddenly the glass table cracked and Mindy, crayon in hand, plunged through the glass with the heels of her hands and her wrists first.

Frightened by the tremendous crash, both children screamed. When blood began to spurt from both of Mindy's forearms, splashing all over the concrete, the shrieking grew louder.

Mindy tried to keep her head. The pain wasn't too bad but the fall had knocked the wind out of her. "I'm okay," she said, for the children and for herself. "Mommy's all right." She looked at the children and was relieved when both appeared terrified but uninjured.

But I'm not, she realized, seeing the great gushes of blood from her arms. All but ignoring the screaming children, she tried to get to her feet but she couldn't get her left hand to do what her brain was telling it to. Some fingers moved, but her wrist wouldn't flex or hold her weight. Leaning on her right elbow, she struggled to a standing position and, leaving great bloody handprints on the door, staggered into the house. "Follow!" she snapped, at that moment more concerned about herself than her panicked children. Still screaming, the two children followed their mother into the house.

She got to the kitchen phone and lifted the receiver with three limp fingers of her right hand, then dropped it onto the kitchen counter. She breathed a sigh of relief when she finally managed to press the digits 9-1-1 with her right index finger. Then, leaving bright red streaks all over the counter, she lifted the receiver.

"9-1-1. What's your emergency?"

"I'm cut. Badly," she shouted over the howls of her children.

"I can't hear you," the operator said.

"Ambulance," she shouted. "Fast."

"Is this the Okamura residence, at 2313 Bayberry Court?"

"Yes," Mindy yelled.

"You need an ambulance?"

"Yes!"

"Okay, I'm dispatching it now. What's the nature . . . ?"

Mindy thanked God that help was on the way and dropped the phone back into its cradle. Then she lifted it again, pressed one of the speed-dial buttons, and said a small prayer.

"Hello?"

"Fran, it's Mindy. Help."

Fran Marterano stood in her kitchen, momentarily paralyzed by the sounds of the wailing children she heard through the receiver. She had never heard such screaming, nor had Mindy ever called her for help like this. "Should I call someone?" she said, totally brain-fogged.

"Come. Please."

"Be right there." She grabbed her own children, three-year-old Sam and five-year-old Tommy, by their wrists and half carried, half dragged them across the back lawn to the Okamura house. As they arrived at the patio, they saw the sprays of blood all over the broken table, the concrete, and the back door. Both boys started to cry. "Is someone dead?" Tommy asked, sobbing.

"You two just be silent," Fran snapped. "Now!"

The two boys sniffled but the noise stopped. Fran opened the back door and charged into the kitchen. She was greeted by the two screaming Okamura children. "You two be silent," Tommy yelled. "Now!"

That's my boy, Fran thought. "Are you hurt?" she asked the children, who had quieted, reacting almost immediately to her son's order. The phone was ringing but Fran ignored it.

"Mommy's hurt," Babs said, starting to cry again.

"Okay. You all stay here. No one goes out of this room. Where's Mommy?" she asked John.

Rubbing his nose, John said, "She went in there. There's blood everywhere."

"Stay here!" Fran followed the bloody trail in search of Mindy.

I was at headquarters posting information about an EMT refresher course I was teaching. In our state, emergency medical technicians must refresh their skills every three years. We take both written and practical skills tests and learn about new equipment and anything that's changed in the state protocols—the prescribed ways of handling emergency situations. As I was standing in the hall, staring at the bulletin board, the klaxon sounded.

"Fairfax Police to Fairfax Ambulance. The rig is needed for a child injured at 2313 Bayberry Court."

"10–4. The ambulance is responding to 2313 Bayberry Court. Will you please page out for an EMT to meet us at the scene?"

I poked my head into the kitchen. "I'll go," I said.

"Great, Joan," Marge Talbot said, keying the mike. "Cancel the page," she told the police. "We've got a full crew." She turned to me, sniffling. "I have a bit of a scratchy throat and I don't want to do patient care if I can avoid it. If you don't mind, will you be crew chief?"

"Sure," I said. "No problem." Most of us in the Fairfield Volunteer Ambulance Corps (FVAC) are both drivers and EMTs.

Marge jumped behind the wheel and Tim Babbett, who had not yet finished his EMT course and was not twenty-one and therefore not old enough to drive the ambulance, climbed into the back. I pressed the button to raise the garage doors and, when the rig was clear, pressed the one to close it. Then I climbed into the passenger seat, and we sped toward Bayberry Court.

"Fairfax Police to rig responding. Just to let you know, when the call came in I heard children screaming. I tried to call back and first got a busy signal and now I get no answer. This might be anything so just wait for our officer who's responding with a short delay."

"Do you suspect an intruder?" I asked. We had to be mindful of our own safety.

"Just stay in the driveway until our officer arrives."

"10–4." Waiting can be the most frustrating part of EMS work. If the police car wasn't already on location, and we weren't sure of the situation, we would just have to cool our heels until it arrived. But it was necessary; we weren't about to rush in to an unknown situation.

We turned onto Bayberry and I checked the house numbers on the mailboxes. As usual, only a few were properly numbered. "This is 2240," I said, "so it's on that side, probably around that bend." I turned to the opening in the back of the rig. "Tim, hand me a pair of gloves and grab the pede bag." The pediatric trauma bag has many of the common supplies, some in smaller sizes specifically designed for working with children. We had everything from tiny BP cuffs and oxygen masks to stuffed animals.

Marge slowed. "2282," I said. "2302." We rounded the bend and saw a woman waving frantically. "That must be it." Marge pulled into the driveway and we climbed out.

"She's hurt really bad," the woman shouted. "She put her hands through a glass table and there's blood everywhere."

"How old's the child?"

"It's not a child. It's the mother."

Marge keyed the mike. "FVAC to FPD. We have a woman injured by glass."

"10–4," the police dispatcher said.

"Tim," I said, grabbing the small trauma bag from the side compartment of the ambulance, "put the pede bag back and get extra trauma dressings and oxygen and follow us."

"Sure thing," Tim said, climbing back into the rear of the ambulance.

"Where?" I asked the woman.

"Inside."

When we opened the front door, the sight was horrendous. I seldom notice the particular decor of houses I respond to, other than to get an overall picture of the living conditions and make a quick assessment to determine any problems we might encounter in getting the patient to the ambulance. The contrast in this hallway and living room was striking. The entire color scheme was white and black. The hall floor had white tile, the living room rug and most of the furniture was white as well. A giant wall unit, the lamps, and tables, throw pillows, and picture frames were black with silver accents.

But now everything was splashed with red. There were blood splotches and splatters on everything, making the scene look like something out of a slasher movie. A small, dazed-looking woman lay in the middle of the living-room floor, with what had once been white towels wrapped around both forearms. The towels were soaked with blood.

"If you don't need me," the woman who had greeted us said, "I'll see to the children."

I became aware of the bedlam coming from the kitchen. "They aren't hurt?"

"No," she said, "just scared."

I nodded and, as she scurried off, walked into the living room. "What happened?" I asked, sitting on the floor beside the tiny woman, knowing my clothes were now bloody. Her yellow T-shirt was soaked, her face was pale and sweaty, and she was trembling.

"I don't know," she said softly. "The table just gave way. I can't seem to make my left hand work."

"Did you fall? Hit your head?"

"No. Just my arms." She looked at her arms, now resting across her abdomen.

"Okay, try to relax and let me have a look." As I peered at the blood-soaked towels, I asked, "What's your name?"

"Mindy Okamura."

"I'm Joan, Mindy." The towel around her right forearm was streaked with blood, but it didn't seem to be getting any redder so I hoped that the bleeding might already be controlled. The body is an amazing machine and usually takes very good care of itself. I looked more carefully at her left arm. Blood had soaked through the layers of towels and was dripping from her elbow. I raised her arm, unwound all but the bottommost layer, what had once been a black-and-white striped kitchen towel, and tried to locate the source of the bleeding. Although I wanted to determine the extent and exact location of the lacerations, I wasn't going to unwrap dressings that might be helping blood to clot.

I glanced at Mindy's pale face then looked up at Marge. "Can you get a quick set of vitals? Use her right arm. I need to keep pressure on this one."

"Okay," she said. Tim arrived with a handful of large trauma dressings. I also saw Police Officer Chuck Harding heading for the kitchen, where the noise of children had eased somewhat.

"Tim, gloves," I said, noting that his hands were bare. "First, open several of those and hand them to me."

Tim unwrapped three 5-by 9-inch thick pads and put them in my hand. I placed them over the towel and pressed hard with both hands, fingers widely spread, holding her arm straight up in the air. Direct pressure and elevation usually work to control all but the most serious bleeding. In Mindy's case, however, I could feel the dressing getting warm with her blood. "Just hold still while I get this bleeding to stop," I said to the frightened woman.

"What about the children?" she asked.

"The woman who was at the end of the driveway is with them, and so's Officer Harding."

She gave me a weak smile. "Fran's a good lady."

Marge said, "BP's 130 over 80, her pulse is 120, and her respirations are about 20."

The signs indicated that Mindy was in early shock, not unexpected from the extent of the bleeding. But so far, at least, her body was compensating for the tremendous loss of blood. "Marge, elevate her feet," I said. "Tim, can you try to find the pressure point in Mindy's arm?"

Tim, his hands now gloved, nodded, crouched beside me, and took Mindy's upper arm.

"You're still bleeding," I said to her, "so we're going to use a pressure point to stop it. Tim's going to press on the main artery that supplies blood to this arm and slow down the flow."

Tim placed the ends of his fingers on the inside of Mindy's left arm and pressed. If the lacerations were reasonably neat, between Tim's pressure and mine and the body's natural abilities, the bleeding would be controlled quickly.

Marge had piled several pillows from the sofa on the floor and placed Mindy's feet on them to help her circulation. "Marge, check her other arm." I looked at our patient. "You've met Tim and Marge and, as I said, I'm Joan." I smiled. "We're going to take good care of you."

Mindy looked up at me. "I'm really scared. Something's wrong with my wrist too. I can't seem to make my hand work right."

"I understand. Try to stay as calm as you can."

"Her right arm seems to be okay," Marge said as she placed a trauma dressing over the towel and wrapped tape around Mindy's arm to limit any additional bleeding when we moved her. "The bleeding's under control."

That was good news, but I could still feel warmth under my fingers and was sure that the bleeding in her left arm wasn't stopping. "Tim, do you have the brachial pulse?" That was the one in Mindy's upper arm, the one Tim should be pressing against.

I watched Tim release his fingers. "Yeah. I've got it," he said, then he reapplied pressure to the brachial artery.

"Marge, let's put Mindy on some oxygen, then get Chuck to help you. I saw him go into the kitchen. Get the stretcher and let's get Mindy out of here." To Tim I said, "Keep the pressure on and let's see whether that will control this bleeding. Hold this dressing a minute with your other hand."

"Can I help?" Mindy asked.

"I want you to just try to relax. We're going to give you a little oxygen. That will help your body cope." Marge hooked the non-rebreather mask to the oxygen cylinder and fitted the mask over Mindy's face.

Tim kept one hand on Mindy's upper left arm and held the dressing with the other while I found more dressings in the trauma bag. Blood was now running down Mindy's upper arm, further soaking the sleeve of the bright yellow Mickey Mouse T-shirt she was wearing. If we weren't able to stop this bleeding, she was going to be in big trouble.

"How are you feeling, Mindy?" I asked, placing more dressings over the ones already in place and reapplying pressure to the wounds.

"Not so good now. I'm a bit dizzy and nauseous. And I'm really shaky."

"I would be too if my arms were injured, but that oxygen should help."

It took only a minute for Marge to return with the stretcher. Without releasing pressure on either the pressure point or the dressings on Mindy's arm, we lifted her onto the stretcher.

"Guys," I said, staring at the blood, which had now soaked through the newest dressings, "I think we need a tourniquet. I can't see any other way. This bleeding isn't slowing down, despite Tim's holding the pressure point. Let's get her into the rig and get another set of vitals."

Awkwardly, trying to maintain as much pressure as we could, we transferred the stretcher to the back of the ambulance and locked it into place. Marge took another set of vitals. "Her blood pressure's now 100 over 70, her pulse rate's"—she paused—"38 times 4 is 142, and her respirations are about 28."

"Joan," Tim said, "we just finished our lecture about this in EMT class, and the instructor suggested using a BP cuff as a tourniquet. It allows you to stop the blood flow just to the injury with as little additional damage as possible."

I thought about it for a moment, then said, "Let's try it."

"Am I in bad shape?" Mindy asked.

"You've lost quite a bit of blood. But we're doing our best to help you." I turned to Marge. "Let's get going to FGH. Tim and I can handle it back here."

"Fairfax General and not St. Luke's? The trauma center has a microsurgery unit."

"I know," I said to Marge. "But she really needs to be stabilized first."

"You got it," Marge said, climbing out the back to go around to the driver's seat.

Tim wrapped a blood pressure cuff around Mindy's left upper arm and squeezed the bulb. "I'll pump this up to about 50 and see whether that works," he said. "That's well below her systolic blood pressure, but it might be enough."

I looked at our patient. "Mindy, we're going to use this blood pressure cuff to try to stop this bleeding. It may make your fingers tingle, but it's supposed to do that." To Tim I said, "Get one more BP before you do that."

As Tim took another blood pressure reading, I removed the outer layer of dressings and applied a fresh white layer so I could see whether Tim's idea was working.

In the past, tourniquets were used as a matter of course for any severe bleeding. Then it was noticed that many soldiers who had been stabilized died shortly after the blood-flow-restricting band was loosened. It was discovered that toxins built up in the uncirculating blood in the limb. When the tourniquet was released, the toxins would circulate through the body, often killing the patient.

EMT protocols now state that a tourniquet is to be used only for life-threatening bleeding, and once it has been applied, EMTs never loosen it. I would have to assess how much danger Mindy was in and decide whether a tourniquet was appropriate, a truly difficult decision. I also had to consider putting on the MAST (military anti-shock trousers) to try to compensate for her decreasing blood pressure, but that could wait. It would take both Tim and me to apply the pressure garment to Mindy's lower body, it would cause Mindy great mental stress, and we had more important things to do.

"Her BP's down to 95 over 70."

Mindy's condition was deteriorating quickly. "Do it," I said. Tim inflated the blood pressure cuff to 50.

I watched the center of the trauma dressing quickly turn red. "Let's pump that up a bit more," I suggested, and Tim inflated the BP cuff to 70. As I watched, the expansion of the red area seemed to slow. As the rig pulled out of the driveway, toward FGH, Marge yelled, "Code 3?"

"Yes, ma'am," I said. I looked at Mindy, her face now white and drenched in sweat. "Let's not waste any time, right, Mindy?"

"Right," she said softly.

I added another layer of snowy-white dressing and watched. Except for a very small area in the center, the gauze remained white. "You know, this is looking good," I said. "I think the bleeding has almost stopped. This was a great idea, Tim."

Tim beamed. "I was afraid I was butting in."

"Not in the least. If you have a good idea, suggest it. I always appreciate help. Let's get another BP."

Tim took another BP cuff, wrapped it around Mindy's right upper arm, and took her blood pressure. "I still get 95 over 70."

"Great," I said. "It's not dropping." I transferred Mindy's oxygen supply from the portable to the main onboard tank, then shifted to the crew chair. I asked her some basic information and noted that her responses hadn't become any more tentative or confused. I entered the data on the prehospital care report, then checked her hands. "Mindy, wiggle your fingers for me."

I watched as her fingers moved. "Good." Then I pressed her right thumb. "Can you feel this?"

"Yes."

I pressed her left. "And this?"

"Yes, but it's fuzzy."

"That's great." Usually I would have a patient squeeze my hands to check grip strength, but I didn't want her arm muscles moving and possibly restarting the bleeding. If I had time before we reached the hospital I might even splint her left arm. I pressed the radio keys to call the hospital. "This is 45–01 to Fairfax ER."

"ER on. Go ahead, 45–01."

"We are en route to your location with a thirty-two-year-old female, a patient of Dr. Osborne. Her arms went through a glass table and both forearms are badly lacerated. She has sensation in her fingers but some impairment of function in the left hand. Bleeding in the right arm was under control prior to our arrival, but we've had difficulty controlling the bleeding in the left. We have a BP cuff inflated to about 70 as a tourniquet and it seems to be working. At ten-fifteen her vitals were"—I checked my notes—"BP 130 over 80, pulse 120, respirations 20. At ten twenty-four her BP was 95 over 70, pulse 142, and respirations 28. It seems to have stabilized now. Our ETA is about three minutes."

"Room one on arrival," the voice from the ER said.

They understood from my communication that this was really serious, and they were putting Mindy in the major trauma cubicle.

"10–4. Room one."

We rode to the hospital in silence, the sound of the siren blaring. As we backed into the ER bay, Tim took another BP. "It's still 95 over 70."

"That's good news, Mindy. Your blood pressure's holding nicely."

We pulled the stretcher from the back of the ambulance and wheeled Mindy through the electronic doors and into cubicle one. "Holy shit," a voice whispered as we passed.

I looked around at the tableau we made. Mindy, Tim, and I were all covered with blood, and the stretcher was soaked around Mindy's left shoulder. We looked like a war zone, and maybe we were one.

With Tim at my side, I gave another complete report to Dr. Morrison. "I wasn't too comfortable about the BP cuff," I said, "but I couldn't think of anything else. Direct pressure, elevation, and the pressure point weren't working and I had to stop the bleeding."

"It seems to have worked, and that's what matters. We'll worry about the rest later. Nice job, guys." He turned to Mindy. "Are you in much pain?"

"Actually, no. It hurts but I can deal with it."

"Good girl. Okay. Let's have a look."

"Doctor," a nurse said, "do you want me to remove this BP cuff?"

"Not on your life," he said. "Just leave it and let's see what we've got." Slowly Dr. Morrison removed the layers of blood-soaked dressings until he got down to the kitchen towel. He looked at me and nodded. I knew he was acknowledging that we hadn't removed the innermost layer. "This might hurt," he said, "but it's wet enough that it should come off easily."

Slowly he peeled the towel off. The sight that greeted us caused one nurse to gasp. Marge walked into the cubicle and we all stared at Mindy's arm. It was in shreds. Long lacerations ran from her wrist to her elbow, and her skin and several layers beneath were in tatters. In several places white bands of ligaments and areas of bone were clearly visible. But there was no bleeding. "You did quite a job on this, ma'am," Dr. Morrison said. "If you had cut crosswise your body would have taken care of the bleeding pretty much by itself, but since the lacerations run the long way, it was impossible for the body to fight it alone. These guys," he continued, motioning to Tim, Marge, and me, "did real good." While I watched, he unwrapped her other arm. As I had suspected, the damage was serious but not as extensive.

"Oh, yes," Mindy said. "Thank you so much. I was so scared, but you really helped me."

"You're welcome," I said. "I'm glad we could help."

Dr. Morrison looked down. "And your name?"

"Mindy Okamura."

He checked the movement in Mindy's right hand. "Well, Mindy, I won't lie to you. You've got some pretty bad lacerations here and we're going to have to do some tests before we can remove this cuff. Then what we'll do is stabilize you here really quickly with lots of intravenous fluids and some blood, then send you down to the trauma center. They have geniuses there who will do whatever's necessary to fix up this hand. You'll probably have quite a bit of physical therapy, but I think you're going to be okay. I can't be positive and everything will be up to the doctors at St. Luke's, but I'm pretty sure."

"Marge has gone to start cleaning up the back of the rig," Tim said as we walked out of the cubicle. "It's a disaster area. Did the doc really say we did okay?"

"We did great," I said, "and, thanks to your idea about the BP cuff, so did Mindy."

"Wow."

"Yeah. Wow. So let's get started cleaning up the equipment. We'll be here at least an hour." Tim was humming as he went looking for the disinfectant to wash the stretcher and the entire inside of the ambulance.

We found out months later that, although she was still undergoing physical therapy, Mindy eventually would regain full use of both hands.

Welcome to Fairfax and the neighboring town of Prescott. These two suburban towns are about fifty miles north of a large city, and over the next three hundred or so pages you're going to spend a lot of time there.

My name is Joan Lloyd and I've been a member of the Fairfax Volunteer Ambulance Corps for about twelve years. I also recently joined the Fire Department Rescue Squad in nearby Prescott. My coauthor and partner, Ed Herman, has been in emergency medical work far longer than I have. He's been with FVAC for more than twenty-five years and with the Prescott rescue squad for almost four years.

We work with wonderful, devoted people, willing to volunteer time and energy to help members of our community. We treat older people with heart attacks, difficulty breathing, and strokes; children with high fevers and broken bones; adults with allergic reactions—people of all ages with the countless and diverse problems encountered by the residents of any town or city. We also respond to serious and nonserious accidents that can happen at any time to anyone.

The people we treat differ as much as people can. My mother always said that when sick or in trouble, people are whatever they are, only more so. It's so true. The sweet, wonderful people become even nicer and the cranky, nasty folks are difficult to deal with. But deal with them we do.

The towns of Fairfax and Prescott are fictional as are all the stores, businesses, and streets within them. We have based the Fairfax Volunteer Ambulance Corps and Prescott's Fire Department Rescue Squad on agencies with which we are affiliated, and we have created Fairfax General Hospital and St. Luke's Trauma Center as representations of a small community hospital and a large, level-1 trauma center, respectively. All the situations are based on calls we have responded to or calls that friends and colleagues have described to us, but we have fictionalized them to protect the privacy of everyone involved. Although emergency medicine changes quickly, the local protocols—our "rules of treatment"—are based on what was in force at the time of the call.

The patients, like Mindy, are fictitious as are all the members of the two emergency medical agencies, the police and fire departments, and other ancillary services. No actual person is portrayed.

The Fairfax Volunteer Ambulance Corps is a basic life-support organization, staffed by EMTs like Ed and me. We can bandage and splint, administer oxygen, do CPR, and use our defibrillator to try to restart a stopped heart. We're specialists in safely caring for victims of auto accidents and unusual emergencies like Mindy's.

Prescott's Volunteer Fire Department Rescue Squad has recently added the services of full-time paid paramedics to their volunteer emergency services. In addition to the basic EMT skills, paramedics can start intravenous lines, administer drugs, and use intubation to keep a patient's airway open in times of critical injury or illness.

Although the actual agencies we ride with have dozens of volunteers, we've simplified the squads for you, using only a limited number of EMTs and paramedics on the calls. If you're curious about them, we've listed all of them at the end of this book. We've also listed the pertinent members of the fire and police departments as well as the staff at the local hospitals to which we transport our patients.

Every vocation has its jargon, and EMS is no exception. We've tried to define each term when it's first used, but if you get puzzled, we've also included a glossary at the back of the book.

So sit back and read about what it's like to respond to ambulance calls as Ed and I do and get to know all the people of Fairfax and Prescott.

Chapter 2

Steve Youngman clung to the side of the pool. He had done thirty laps and was finished with his workout for the day. He rested as he thought about how good the sauna would feel. Just the thing to take the ache out of his arms and shoulders. As he idly watched the young woman in the next lane swim past, he suddenly realized that something was wrong. She was facedown in the water but she had stopped making any forward progress. Her arms and legs seemed to be thrashing randomly. Then, without a sound, she sank to the bottom of the pool. Steve had been an EMT in the city for many years, and he reacted instantly. He dove to the bottom just as Penny Harris, the health club lifeguard, saw what was happening and jumped into the water. Within a few moments, Steve and Penny brought the woman to the surface and got her out of the pool.

"Are you all right?" Penny yelled as she knelt next to the woman who lay on her back staring at the ceiling.

The woman did not respond. Penny placed her cheek next to the woman's mouth, listening for breathing and watching her chest for movement. She simultaneously placed her index and middle fingers at the side of the woman's neck, feeling for a pulse. "She's not breathing,

20

but I have a good carotid pulse," she said, looking up at Steve. "I'll start rescue breathing. Go call 911."

"Okay, I'll be right back." Steve dashed toward the telephone as Penny began to blow into the woman's mouth.

Joan and I were trying to find excuses to avoid going to the Prescott Health Club to work out. "Ed, I've really got too much work to do today," Joan said. "And besides, the escalator at the mall was broken this morning and I had to walk up to the second floor. That counts as aerobic exercise, doesn't it?"

"Yeah, sure," I replied. "And I've got a headache. Working out will probably make it worse. Maybe I'll just skip today and do a longer workout tomorrow." We gave each other our who-do-you-think-you're-kidding look just as the pager tones went off.

"GVK–861 Prescott to the rescue squad. A full crew is needed for the ambulance to respond to 111 Bark Street for a woman having a seizure. Will a full crew please call in. GVK–861 Prescott, clear."

"That's the health club," Joan said. "I guess God wants us to work out today."

I grabbed the phone and dialed the firehouse. "It's Ed Herman," I said. "Joan and I will respond to the scene. Just get a driver to bring the rig."

Joan and I dashed out of the house, jumped into my car, and drove toward the club with the blue light flashing as the pager beeped again. "GVK–861 Prescott to the rescue squad. A driver is needed for a call at the Prescott Health Club. Please call in. GVK–861, clear."

"If it's just a seizure she'll probably be okay by the time we get there. She'll probably RMA," I said as we headed toward the club. Most seizures are self-limiting, and the patient usually revives and refuses medical attention. But was this really a seizure?

Joan looked at me doubtfully and I understood her thoughts without anything being said. We had responded to three cardiac arrests at the club in the past two years. For a "health" club, things sometimes didn't seem very healthy there.

"GVK–861 Prescott to all units responding to Bark Street. CPR is in progress at that location," the pager announced.

"Oh, shit," Joan and I said simultaneously.

"As soon as we pull up, you go in," I said to Joan. "I'll get the BVM out of the trunk and follow." Neither of us wanted to do mouth-to-mouth, and the bag-valve mask resuscitator would be more efficient anyway.

As we approached the club I could see a police car with its trunk open standing in front of the entrance. "That's Mike Gold's patrol car," Joan said. "He'll have a BVM with him. Don't bother with yours."

I pulled up behind the police car, and Joan and I sprinted into the club. One of the employees met us at the door. "Over there," she said, pointing toward the pool. As we entered the pool area, I could see Mike Gold kneeling at the head of a supine woman, holding the mask of the bag-valve-mask resuscitator against her mouth, rhythmically squeezing the large rubber bag to force 100 percent oxygen into her lungs. A woman in a swimsuit was doing chest compressions. A tall man whom I recognized as an EMT who had ridden with FVAC years before was standing next to them. I walked over to the man.

"Steve. What happened?" I asked.

"Penny and I pulled her out of the pool and started CPR," he said.

"Was she diving? Did she hit her head?"

"No. She was just swimming. She seemed to convulse and then she sank like a stone."

I looked down at the woman. "You guys are doing a great job. Her color is still really good." I knelt next to Mike. "Do you want me to relieve you?"

"Yeah, okay, Ed," Mike replied, handing me the BVM.

"Stop CPR," I said to Penny, and placed my cheek next to the woman's face and felt for a pulse in her neck. "Okay, let's continue CPR. She's not breathing and she has no pulse."

I placed the mask over the woman's nose and mouth, made a "C" with my left thumb and index finger, and hooked my left ring finger under her jaw to apply counter-pressure and make a good seal with the mask. Then I began to squeeze the bag with my right hand. Joan took over chest compressions.

Within a few minutes paramedics Amy Chen and Hugh Washington arrived. They attached the leads of a cardiac monitor—two under the collarbones and one under the left rib—to the woman's body.

"Stop CPR," Amy said.

We all looked at the flat line that was displayed on the screen of the monitor. "She's in asystole. Continue CPR," Amy said.

While Joan and I did CPR, Hugh started an IV line and Amy intubated the woman—inserted a tube into her trachea to assure a good airway. I could then squeeze the oxygen bag attached to the tube without having to keep a seal with the mask. Hugh injected one milligram each of epinephrine and atropine into a port in the IV line.

"Stop CPR," he ordered.

Joan and I stopped and glanced hopefully at the cardiac monitor, but it still showed a flat line. "Continue CPR," Hugh told us. After three more minutes of CPR, Hugh injected two more milligrams of epinephrine into the IV line. "Stop CPR," Hugh said. This time we could all see the jagged peaks that indicated cardiac activity on the monitor screen. "Check for a pulse," Hugh said. "The monitor is showing a good rhythm."

Joan reached out to the woman's neck while I felt her wrist just below the thumb. "She has a strong carotid pulse," Joan said, amazed. It's always a fantastic feeling when we are able to restore a heart's regular beat.

"And a weak radial also," I added as I felt the artery at the thumb side of her wrist pulse under my fingers. A sigh of relief went through the group that was struggling so hard to save the woman's life. As I looked down, however, I could see that she still was not breathing so I continued to squeeze oxygen into her lungs. I was also discouraged by the fact that, despite the brightness of the pool area, the woman's pupils were widely dilated.

"Let's get a BP," Hugh said.

Brenda Frost, who had arrived with the ambulance, took a blood pressure reading. "Seventy-two over 40," she reported.

"That's great," Hugh said. "Let's move her."

Within minutes, as I continued to bag her, we rolled the woman onto a backboard, placed her on a stretcher, and loaded her into the ambulance. In the ambulance, however, although the cardiac monitor showed what appeared to be a normal heart rhythm, both her radial and carotid pulses disappeared. I glanced at Hugh. "EMD?" I asked.

"Yeah," Hugh confirmed. "You guys had better start CPR again." Although the electrical activity of the woman's heart appeared to be normal, those impulses were not triggering any beating, a condition known as electromechanical dissociation. She was again in cardiac arrest.

Hugh now administered three milligrams of epinephrine and we stopped to check for pulses again.

"I have a fast pulse," Joan said, palpating the woman's neck. The monitor showed a rapid but normal-appearing heart rhythm.

I moved my fingers around at the base of the woman's thumb, trying to find a radial pulse. "Nothing," I said, glancing at Hugh.

"See if you can get a BP," he suggested.

We had left the BP cuff deflated but still wrapped around the woman's arm. While Joan continued bagging her, I placed the diaphragm of my stethoscope on the inside of her elbow—over the brachial artery—and inflated the cuff to a pressure of 200 milligrams of mercury. I cracked the valve and listened and watched the needle of the pressure indicator as the cuff slowly deflated. I heard nothing through the earpieces of the stethoscope as the needle steadily went down to zero. "She has no recordable blood pressure," I said.

"Okay," Hugh said. "Her heart is beating. Now let's see if we can get her BP up." He opened the valve on the IV line so that normal saline solution began rapidly flowing into the woman's body. Within a few minutes I could feel a pulse at the base of her thumb.

"I've got a radial," I announced as I inflated the BP cuff again. This time I didn't use the stethoscope. I just kept my finger on the spot where I had felt the radial pulse, while I allowed the cuff to deflate. As the falling pressure-gauge needle passed 104, I suddenly felt a pulse. "I've got a BP of 104 by palp," I reported.

"That's great," Hugh said. "It looks like we have a viable patient."

Although our patient never breathed on her own or regained consciousness, we delivered her to Fairfax General Hospital with a good heartbeat. It had been a good "save," but would she live? And if she did live, would it be as a "vegetable"?

The next day I learned that the woman had had a ruptured aneuryism—a swollen blood vessel had burst in her brain. She was still alive but in a coma. It was discouraging. More often than not, cardiac arrest victims do not make it, despite all our efforts, but we always hope for a miracle. It looked like this wasn't going to be one.

The following day, while bringing a victim of a minor motor vehicle accident into the emergency room, I saw Dr. Margolis, the head of the ER, doing some paperwork. After delivering my patient and finishing my report, I walked over to him. "Hi, Doc. How did the woman with the aneuryism make out?" I asked, not really wanting to hear the answer.

Dr. Margolis was obviously intent on his work. "Oh, she's still alive but her EEG is flatline," he said, not looking up from his writing.

The woman's brain was dead. "Yeah, I figured as much," I said. "I guess all that effort was a waste."

Dr. Margolis looked up at me and put his pen down. "Wait a minute, Ed," he said. "Everyone who cared for her before she got here did a great job. You got her here in good physical condition except for her brain, which

was pretty much destroyed as soon as her aneuryism ruptured. She never had a chance at recovery, no matter what
anyone might have done. And what you did wasn't a
waste.

"Since her body was alive and in good condition, we
have had time to get permission from her family and
we're making the necessary arrangements to harvest her
organs. We're keeping her blood circulating until we can
get everything in place. That wouldn't have been possible if she had been dead when you brought her in. Yes,
you lost one patient, but you saved the life of the person
who will get her heart and the person who will get her
liver and the people who will get her kidneys. And
maybe a blind person will see again through her eyes.
The people who started CPR and your rescue squad
saved a number of lives this time, and you should be very
proud."

Stunned, I stood rooted to the spot for a few seconds as
I digested what I had been told. "Thanks, Doc," I said,
then slowly walked out to where the ambulance waited to
bring me home, or to the next call.

My name is Ed Herman and I'm an EMT. I'm also a
biologist and a writer, but, even though I don't get paid
for my emergency medical work, being an EMT is the
job that is most satisfying to me. In previous books I've
written about some of my reasons for becoming an EMT,
such as my fantasy of rescuing beautiful young women in
distress. But human motivations are rarely simple. It
seems that I always wanted to know enough to be able to
help people in emergency medical situations. I especially
remember the time when my father got burned.

As a kid, I spent my summers in the Maine resort town

of Old Orchard Beach. It was a child's wonderland—a broad beach with fine, white sand and a number of amusement parks. We lived in a small cottage behind the restaurant my father owned. I am told that, when I was very young, I often wandered away from home. My parents were never very concerned, however, because they knew where to find me. I would always be on the merry-go-round, where the operator would let me ride for free. Times were different fifty years ago. Everyone in town knew my parents and would look out for me, and my mother knew it. So, when she realized that I was missing, she would simply stroll over to the merry-go-round and take me home.

As far back as I can remember I was self-employed during my summers in Old Orchard Beach. I would comb the beach daily collecting soda bottles, which I would return for deposits. Then I would spend my earnings on amusement park rides or on pinball machines. I was a "pinball wizard" and often could parlay a nickel into enough free games to keep myself entertained for an entire afternoon.

One of my favorite times in Old Orchard was the evening, after the dinner "rush" was over. My father would remove his apron and seat himself in the front booth. To me he was a king holding court. He loved people and delighted in talking to everyone. Anyone who came in was welcome to sit down with him. Many were customers who vacationed in Old Orchard every summer and had known him for years.

There was a theater and dance hall at the end of the pier, where all of the big bands played in the forties and early fifties, and my father's restaurant was the place to go after the show. I was always awed by the famous entertainers who would chat with him. And there were some visitors who were not famous but who seemed to be treated with a great deal of "respect" by those around them—like Benny, a short, somewhat overweight man who was always accompanied by two very large, silent, and expressionless "friends." They never sat down, even when Benny slid into the booth to visit with my father.

I was in my early teens, working behind the counter making sandwiches when the accident happened. Marion, who was working behind the counter with me, had just made a fresh urn of coffee. As she finished and started to move away from the big tank, her apron string snagged on the urn handle and the entire ten-gallon silver tank started to tip. My father, who was standing next to her, saw what was happening. He could have gotten out of the way but instead he pushed Marion to the side, and ten gallons of boiling water poured over one of his legs.

I stood there in a state of shock, with no idea of what to do. One of the customers in the restaurant identified herself as a nurse and took control. She removed my father's pants and I could see that his entire leg was red and blistered, with large flaps of skin hanging off. Then she asked for some flour. I ran into the kitchen and got a bucket of flour, which she proceeded to pour all over my father's leg.

My father was in the hospital for three weeks. At times during those weeks, he was not expected to live because of the massive infection caused by the flour that the "nurse" had poured all over him. But he survived and I was determined never again to be helpless and ignorant in an emergency medical situation. I read as much as I could about first aid, but little information was available at the time. First-aid books were meant primarily for wilderness situations and gave useful information about topics like "how to make a stretcher out of tree branches" and "how to suck the poison out of a snake bite." The science of prehospital medical care had not yet been invented, and ambulances provided transportation but little else. Many years later, after witnessing a terrible motorcycle accident and again feeling that sense of helplessness and frustration at my inability to help, I walked into the headquarters of FVAC and asked, "How do I join FVAC and how do I become an EMT?" I now teach first-aid courses and call one of my favorite lectures "No-Nos in First Aid, or What *Not* to Do Before the Ambulance Arrives."

Chapter 3

Teenagers are a strange breed, neither fish nor fowl nor good red herring, as my grandmother used to say, and there's no way to know how they are going to react in an emergency situation when no parent is around. Sometimes they behave like full-grown, mature adults, and sometimes they become children again. Unfortunately, sometimes in the latter cases, I get involved.

"A full crew is needed for a bicyclist hit by a car on Floral Way, just down from the intersection with Oak Hill," my radio blared.

I keyed my microphone and said, "45–24 to Fairfax Police. I'll respond to the scene." Having just been to the bank and the post office, I was in my car, only a few moments from the location. It was a hot summer Thursday morning and I had all my windows open, enjoying the heat and unusually low humidity.

"10–4." The tones sounded again. "Fairfax Police to all home units. A driver and an attendant are still needed for this accident at Floral Way and Oak Hill. Be advised that EMT Lloyd will meet you at the scene."

I arrived at the intersection, pulled my car over, jumped out, and ran toward the gathered crowd. As I trotted toward the scene, I noticed a ten-speed bike lying in the grass on the side of the road. "I'm with the ambulance," I said, worming my way through the curious throng. I looked over the edge of the eight-foot embankment. There, most of his body in a small slow-flowing stream, was a young man, his face on a rock just out of the water. I climbed down the embankment and got to the boy, trying not to get my jeans and sneakers too wet.

I crouched beside a boy of about twelve or thirteen, dressed in a now-soaked Grateful Dead T-shirt and jean shorts, and used my palms to hold his head still. He was bony and angular, all shoulder blades and knobby knees, the typical shape of a young teenage boy. "Can you hear me?" When I got no response I leaned over and yelled into his ear. "What's your name?" Still no response. Holding his head with one hand, I reached down with the other and pinched a bit of skin on the back of his hand between my nails. He moaned slightly but didn't move.

I examined the boy's body and saw very little damage. No abrasions, no cuts or scratches. Hoping that he wouldn't move and possibly injure his neck, I released my hold on his head and carefully did a full survey to try to ascertain the extent of his injuries. The checkover revealed nothing obvious, and I was becoming increasingly puzzled by his condition. His breathing was very slow and his skin was icy cold. I also noticed a strong smell of alcohol. I carefully examined his head for bleeding, depressions, or any other indication of head injury that might be the cause of his unconsciousness but found nothing.

I took head stabilization again, knowing there was little I could do without help from my crew and equipment from the rig. Although I wanted to get him out of the water so he could warm up, I didn't dare move him without lots of help and a long backboard to put him on. Fortunately, I soon heard the familiar sound of sirens, both police and ambulance. "Did anyone see what happened?" I called up to the crowd of bystanders.

"I think he was hit by a car," one said.

"His bike is lying here beside the road," someone shouted.

"He must have fallen," another cried. "After he was hit."

"The car must have driven off. How could someone have done something like that?"

I tried to get people's attention. "But did anyone actually *see* anything?"

I was greeted with silence. "Someone look at the bike," I said, "and see what part of it is damaged."

After a moment, as both a police car and the ambulance pulled to a stop beside the roadway, someone yelled, "The bike's fine. I don't see any damage at all." Three other people walked to the bike to look and all agreed that there seemed to be no damage to the vehicle.

"Is there a helmet anywhere?" I yelled.

"Not here."

"No, we don't see one."

Then a familiar face appeared over the edge of the embankment. "What do you need, Joan?" Marge Talbot yelled down to me.

"I'm glad to see you, Marge. I need a longboard, collars, straps, and head blocks. And towels to dry him off with, and a blanket."

"Okay. We're coming."

Stan Poritsky, the first police officer to arrive, climbed down to me. "What are his injuries?" he asked.

"I don't really know," I answered. "I haven't found anything obvious. No bleeding or obvious deformity that would indicate broken bones. But he's barely responsive, even to pain."

"Do you smell alcohol?" Stan asked.

"I sure do. But he's only a kid."

"Lots of kids drink," Stan said, and I nodded, not wanting to admit that my patient, a twelve- or thirteen-year-old boy, might be drunk.

Marge and Sam Middleton climbed down the embankment with the equipment I had requested. Careful not to cause any movement of his head and neck, we put on a cervical collar and logrolled the boy onto the long backboard. We quickly strapped him down and taped head blocks in place. Once he was secure, Sam and I used several towels to dry him off. As we prepared to carry him up to the ambulance, I said, "Let's be extra careful moving him. I think he's hypothermic, and movement might throw him into v-fib." The extreme cold of his body might make his heart muscle irritable and thus cause it to contract irregularly, a life-threatening condition.

As gently as possible, Stan, Marge, Sam, and I carried the boy up to the ambulance, put the board onto the stretcher, and lifted it into the ambulance. Then Sam, Marge, and I climbed inside to prepare him for transport to the hospital. I found an oxygen mask, connected it to the onboard supply, and prepared to put it over the boy's face.

But as Marge started to take a set of vitals, the boy moaned, heaved, and started to vomit. "Shit," we all said in unison. When someone is strapped to a spineboard with his head firmly secured with head blocks and tape, it's impossible for him to turn his head to the side when he vomits. It's our job to protect his airway so that no vomited material gets into his lungs. We quickly turned our patient, board and all, on his side and awkwardly supported him there.

While Marge and I held the board, Sam grabbed for the suction tube, but he wasn't fast enough. Soon vomit, smelling strongly of alcohol, covered the floor of the ambulance. While balancing the board on its edge, Marge grabbed several more towels and put them below the boy's mouth while Sam flipped on the suction motor. He pulled off the slender Yankauer tip that allows us to suction blood and mucus from a patient's upper airway and used the half-inch tube, wide open, to try to clean out the boy's mouth.

I watched Sam swallow hard. Around the corps he has a reputation of having a slightly weak stomach. He tells his patients, quite candidly, "You vomit, I vomit."

"We can handle this," I said to him. "Why don't you just get us to FGH. But wait until we can get him back onto the stretcher before you start."

"Bless you," he said, swallowing again, then he climbed out the side door. Over the sounds of the boy's retching, I could hear Sam drawing in lungfuls of fresh air. We all have our weaknesses, I thought. I can't lift anything heavy, but vomit really doesn't bother me.

When the heaving seemed to slow down, we stopped the suction and Marge and I slowly lowered the back-board/boy combination back down onto the stretcher and strapped him down. "What a mess," Marge said. "We'll be cleaning out the back of this rig for an hour."

I sighed, agreeing that it would be at least that long before we could get the rig clean enough to use again.

I wet a towel with sterile water, the only water we

carry, and wiped the boy's face, then put the oxygen mask on him. He moaned, then his eyes opened. "What happened?" he asked softly.

"You're in an ambulance. Do you remember what happened?"

"Bike. Needed a drink so I went down to the water. That's all I remember."

"What's your name, son?" I asked.

"Joseph Priestly, but my friends call me Slick. I'm cold."

I noted that he wasn't shivering. "I can imagine."

Marge had finished taking a set of vitals. "His BP's 90 over 55, his resps are 14 and shallow, and his pulse is 45." All the numbers were very low.

"Tell me what hurts," I asked Slick, noting his slurred speech, probably from the cold.

"Nothing. I'm just real cold." His lowered vital signs and lack of shivering indicated hypothermia to me. I touched his arm and his skin was icy cold. His body's core temperature was probably below ninety degrees, the point at which shivering stops. "Marge, do we have any of those chemical heat packs?"

"Let me take a look," she said.

I looked at the boy. "I think you're extra cold. It's called hypothermia. Have you had anything to drink today? Any alcohol?" When he hesitated, I continued, "It's important for the hospital to know. If they want to give you some medicine that might react badly with alcohol, they need to know whether you've had any."

"Some beers."

"What's some? A beer or two?"

"Or more."

"Like how many?"

"Maybe two sixes." He drifted back to sleep.

"Oh," I said. I turned and yelled to Sam, "Let's go. But take it real easy on the bumps."

"Right. Code 3?" Sam yelled.

"I think so. Let's get him there but go easy." Before he vomits again, I added mentally.

"I got it. Fast but slow," Sam said.

"Right," I said, grinning.

Marge found two heat packs, and we broke the inner container and allowed the two chemicals to mix. I wrapped each hot plastic bag of liquid in a pillowcase and placed one under each of Slick's arms. During the trip to the hospital, Slick awoke a few times and we managed to get his address, phone number, and date of birth. As I had suspected, he was thirteen years old and drunk as a skunk. At least he didn't vomit again.

At Fairfax General, we transferred the boy to the hospital gurney and filled them in on what we knew. It took almost an hour to finish the paperwork and then get the ambulance cleaned up and as sanitized as we could. At headquarters, we would leave the doors open and let the sunlight and fresh air complete the job.

The following morning I brought an eighty-five-year-old woman to FGH. Her daughter had told us that her mother had been complaining that her heart kept stopping, but when I put her on the monitor, I saw a normal rhythm. I had no direct idea what her complaints were since the mother spoke only Hungarian. After we got the older woman loaded, her daughter took off to drive to the hospital in her own car, leaving us alone with the woman who smiled, talked incessantly, and frequently pointed to her chest, unconcerned that no one understood her. Each time she pointed, I listened, but the steady beeping of the monitor indicated no change in her heart activity.

When we had settled our patient in a small cubicle, I saw one of the nurses who had been on duty the previous day. "How's the boy we brought in yesterday, the one who was hypothermic?" I asked.

"You aren't going to believe this," she said. "His core temperature was 89 and his blood alcohol was 2.8."

"That's almost three times the legal limit for DWI," I said, aghast.

She nodded. "I know. He must have been drinking all morning."

I sighed, shook my head, waved good-bye to the Hungarian woman, and climbed back into the ambulance. Oh, well.

The ambulance was dispatched to a man with an allergic reaction to something he ate. There was no duty crew available so when the police paged out, I called in. "Mark," I said when I heard the dispatcher's voice, "I'll respond to the scene."

"Thanks, Joan. Fred Stevens is getting the rig. I'll try for an attendant but I might not be able to get one. It's really deserted today."

"Do what you can, Mark," I said, then headed for my car. It was early spring and the sky had been darkening all afternoon.

The address given was on Old Bridge Road, and it took only a few minutes for me to arrive at the scene. When I pulled into the driveway I saw a man with an oxygen mask on his face sitting on a large rock beside the front walk, Officer Chuck Harding beside him. Despite the cool temperatures, the man was wearing only a tight, short-sleeved black T-shirt, showing off a well-developed upper body, black jeans, and a black baseball cap pulled low over his forehead.

"How are you doing?" I asked as I walked up to him, carrying my crash kit.

"I'm fine now. I have allergies so I used my stick and I'm fine now."

By "stick" I assumed he meant his injectable epinephrine, carried and used by allergic patients to ward off severe reactions. "What caused you to use the epi?" I asked.

"I got stung by a bee. It's nothing."

The dispatch information was partly right anyway. "Where were you stung?"

He grinned. "In the backyard." I raised an eyebrow. "On my arm here." He showed me his arm and a hard, red, hot area just below his elbow.

"How long ago were you stung?"

"About fifteen minutes."

"And how long after did you use the epi?"

"Right away. I'm really fine now. If I don't feel okay later I'll just go to my doctor. I don't want no ambulance."

"You can certainly refuse treatment," I said. "I'm not going to kidnap you. But will you at least let me take some vitals and listen to your lungs?"

"You won't take me anywhere. I'll just go to my doctor later if I need to."

I keyed my microphone and told the rig to proceed with caution, without lights or siren, and indicated that this patient might be an RMA, a refusal of medical attention.

Police dispatcher Mark Thomas called by radio.

"45–24. Be advised I'm unable to get an attendant. Do you want Prescott for mutual aid?"

"No. I think we can handle this."

"10–4."

I looked at the man, who appeared to be about twenty-five, and carefully checked for generalized redness or swelling, hives, or any other signs of an allergic reaction. He looked fine to me, although, since I had never seen him before, I had no way of knowing whether his slightly puffy lips were normal for him. "Sir, your face might be a bit swollen."

"I'm fine. I really don't want you here."

"When the ambulance gets here you can sign our form that declines any treatment, but until then let me listen to your lungs and take vitals."

"If you have to."

I was getting a bit annoyed at the man's macho attitude. There was an I-don't-need-any-help swagger about him that got my back up. "I do," I said, putting on gloves and taking my BP cuff and stethoscope from my kit. I checked his vitals and all were within normal limits. I listened to his lungs and heard a slight whistling. "Are you sure you're all right? Your lungs don't sound completely normal to me. Why don't you let us take you over to the hospital so they can check you over just to be sure?" I asked one last time as I heard the siren.

"No. I'm not going." He pulled off the oxygen mask, dropped it onto the ground, stood up, and began to pace. I unfastened the mask from the officer's oxygen tank and stuffed it into my jacket pocket.

I shrugged. I didn't know whether he needed attention or not. He was the only one who knew. And he certainly had the right to refuse. I wasn't happy about it but I would document everything, have him sign an RMA, then get the police officer to witness his signature and let him go on his way.

The ambulance pulled into the driveway and Fred climbed out with the clipboard. It started to drizzle so we suggested that the man get into the ambulance so we could all stay dry. "If I gotta," he said. I sighed and climbed in behind him. We sat side by side on the bench while Fred dropped into the crew seat. "Okay," I said, taking the clipboard, "I need your full name."

"Charles Prosetti."

As I wrote that, I asked his address. "2786 Old Bridge Road, Fairfax," he said and I duly recorded the information.

"Why did you call us if you didn't think you needed treatment?"

"I thought my parents would kill me if I didn't."

"How old are you?" I asked.

"Old enough to know better," he said with a vicious laugh.

Okay. Fine. "Your date of birth, sir?" I could figure his age out later.

"April 23."

"And the year?"

"You don't need that, do you?"

"Yes, sir, I do."

He mumbled something I couldn't understand. "Nineteen eighty?" Fred said.

"Yeah," he grumbled.

"That makes you only seventeen," I said. "I'm afraid we have a problem." Since he was under age, he couldn't legally refuse our help. Parental consent for emergency treatment and transport to the hospital was legally implied and, without the refusal of a parent or guardian, we had to transport him. And from his reluctance to give his age, he obviously knew it. Of course he could have lied and we would have had no way to verify the information, but he had told the truth. I assumed that Mr. Macho wanted to be forced.

"I know," he said. "I don't want to go. I'm fine."

"Is there a parent or someone else around who can refuse for you?"

"No. My folks are on a cruise."

"Older brother or sister, uncle, someone like that?"

"Nah. But I don't want to go with you."

"Unfortunately, we can't let you refuse. You have to be checked at the hospital."

"Come on, lady, let's just say I'm eighteen and let me go."

"I can't. I'll get killed by my captain, the corps' attorney, and everyone else at FVAC." We have no regular attorney but my patient's cooperation would make this all run much more smoothly. If I could get around his I-don't-need-anybody attitude, everything would be easier.

"All right," he grumbled.

"Great," I said brightly. "We can finish this paperwork while Fred gets us to the hospital. Who's your doctor?"

"I don't go to any."

"Someone gave you the prescription for the epi stick," I said.

He sighed. "Marconi."

I knew Dr. Marconi slightly and I had transported several of his patients to FGH. "Fairfax General? That's where Marconi is."

"Sure, whatever."

I sighed. I ascertained that he was allergic to bee stings

and nothing else that he knew of. He had no other medical conditions I needed to document. "How's your breathing?" I asked, writing the vitals I had already obtained on the PCR.

"It's okay."

"Just okay?" I pressed, remembering the whistles I had heard. "How about some oxygen?"

"If I've got to."

Everything was going to be a battle. Trying to sound cheerful, I said, "It might be a good idea." I got out a non-rebreather oxygen mask and connected it to the main oxygen supply.

As Fred got into the driver's seat, I said, "And how about shifting over onto the stretcher? It will be more comfortable and I can seat belt you in there."

"I ain't lying down like no patient."

"You can sit up if you like," I said, adjusting the back of the stretcher. Grudgingly he moved to the stretcher and put his legs up. Then I helped him fasten the seat belts and adjust the oxygen mask over his face.

Since he didn't want to talk during the ride, I took the time to begin writing the assessment section of the PCR. About halfway to FGH, I said, "I'm going to call the hospital and let them know we're coming. I want you to listen and make sure I get all the information right." I pressed the numbered keys to set off the tones in Fairfax General's Emergency Room. "45–01 to Fairfax ER."

A moment later a voice came through the radio. "FGH on. Go ahead, 45–01."

"We are en route to your location with a seventeen-year-old victim of a bee sting. He's a patient of Dr. Marconi. He took an epi stick approximately twenty minutes ago. He claims to have no symptoms but his face is a bit swollen and I heard some wheezing in both lungs. His vitals are pulse 76 and regular, respirations 16, BP 122 over 76. Our ETA is five minutes."

"Is there a parent or guardian with you?"

"Negative. He says his parents aren't reachable."

"10–4. We'll await your arrival."

The hospital could try to sort out the authorization for treatment. In a life-threatening emergency, of course, they could treat anyway, so if the allergic reaction became severe they could give the appropriate medications. Whatever happened, I had complete confidence that they would quickly get his condition under control.

As I replaced the microphone in the holder, he said, "I'm getting cold. Got a blanket?"

"Sure," I said, getting him a woolen blanket and covering him with it. As I tucked the blanket around his legs, I noticed that his face was more swollen. "Is your face bothering you? It looks swollen."

"Maybe."

"Would you like a cold pack? It might help the swelling."

"No!"

Yeah. Right. Heaven save me from macho crap. Oxygen and the blanket were about all I could do for him, so I completed the rest of my report. Once we were stopped in the ambulance bay, I listened to his lungs again. The wheezing was louder now. Obviously the epi hadn't been enough to completely stop the reaction.

We wheeled him into the emergency room and into a cubicle. I gave a complete report to Rosemary Harper, the nurse in charge. "I understand you're not eighteen yet, Charles," she said.

"Yeah," he said.

As she began to get information about how the hospital could reach someone able to give consent for treatment, I walked out of the cubicle. I submitted the report and Fred and I remade the stretcher. "Lord, I hate this teenage shit," said Fred, never one to mince words. "Probably afraid his girlfriend would think he was a sissy."

I just rolled my eyes.

It was a beautiful, midsummer Tuesday morning and I was returning to headquarters on 45–01 from a call for a woman in labor. I've delivered two babies in my years with FVAC, and each was such a wonderful experience that I kept hoping to deliver another. Unfortunately for me, but fortunately for the expectant mother, we arrived at the hospital in plenty of time. We were about halfway back to headquarters when the radio squawked. "Fairfax Police to Fairfax Ambulance."

"45–01 on," Stephanie DiMartino said from the shotgun seat. Jack McCaffrey was driving.

"Do you have a full crew on board?"

"10–4," Stephanie said, then released the SEND key and groaned. "We've got another one."

" 'Fraid so," Jack grumbled.

"We need you to respond to Route 10 in front of the middle school for a 10–2."

"10–4," Stephanie said. "Any idea how many injuries?"

"I'll let you know when we get an officer to the scene."

"10–4," Stephanie said as Jack flipped on the emergency lights and siren. "Did you hear?" she yelled over her shoulder to me.

"Yeah. Auto accident. Want gloves?"

When Stephanie reached behind her I handed her a pair of latex gloves for herself and one for Jack. Then I put on a pair myself.

"Fairfax Police to 45–01."

"–01 is on," Stephanie said.

"Officer at the scene says three in the car, all minor injuries, all teenagers."

"Oh, goody," Jack muttered. "Teenage hysterics. I just love it."

We had all experienced the reactions of young people, the ink barely dry on their drivers' licenses, thinking about telling their parents that their shiny new vehicles were being towed to the body shop. I sighed. I'm usually pretty good with kids since I used to teach seventh and eighth grade but . . .

Moments later we arrived at the scene. The car was nowhere in sight and there was a mob of people milling around, including two police officers, several firemen who had come to the scene in case of extrication, and about a dozen teens. We quickly found Officer Eileen Flynn. "What have we got?" I asked.

"Three kids were in the car, all counselors at the day camp here. The boy who was driving and the girl from the backseat are over there. I think they're the only ones injured." She pointed to a knot of kids. Stephanie and Jack headed for the victims. "Joan, would you come over to my car?" Eileen asked. "The third kid, the front seat passenger, is in there. She's uninjured but she's pretty shook up."

I followed Eileen to her patrol car and found a teenage girl seated on the edge of the passenger seat, shaking, with deep rapid respirations. She was crying loudly.

"Okay," I said, putting my arm around her shoulders. "It's okay. You're doing fine. Just try to relax. What's your name?" I asked, hoping to get her attention. She just continued to shake, her head resting on her palms, elbows on her knees.

"I'm sorry. . . . I'm sorry. . . . It's my fault. . . . I'm sorry. . . ." Every phrase was punctuated by deep, heavy breaths.

"What's your name?"

Slowly she raised her eyes and looked at me. "I'm sorry . . . I'm so scared."

I cupped her face and crouched down so I was looking directly into her eyes. "I know you're scared but I need to know your name."

"Missy. Melissa. . . . I'm sorry."

"You were the passenger?"

"Yes." Tears streamed down her face.

"Are you hurt anywhere?"

"No," she said. "But my fingers feel funny."

"I'm sure they do. That's because you're breathing much too fast. I need you to concentrate on slowing your breathing down." When her breathing didn't immediately slow, I repeated, more strongly, "Missy. Slow your breathing down." I moved her face so she was again looking into my eyes. "Slow your breathing down. You can do it. Try to relax. The shaking and the funny feeling in your arms are both because of your fast breathing and your nervousness." Maybe I can get her to focus on something else, I thought, so I pulled a small pad from my pocket. "Give me your full name."

"Melissa Pavone. . . ."

"And your address?"

As she gave me the rest of her information, her

breathing slowed a bit. I quickly palpated her neck, back, and the rest of her body, and found no injuries of any kind. Now came the difficult part. She had to be transported to the hospital since I was pretty sure she was under eighteen. "Missy, how old are you?"

"I'm fifteen." Bingo. She wasn't old enough to refuse treatment so I would have to take her to the hospital, without increasing her anxiety and her breathing rate, I hoped.

"Missy. We're going to take you over to Fairfax General. I have to do this since you're not eighteen yet. You know and I know there's nothing wrong with you, but my rules give me no choice."

"I'm sorry. . . . I'm so upset. . . ."

"I know," I said, listening to her breathing speed up again.

"How's Jen and Mitch? It was his car."

"I don't know how everyone else is. Let's just take care of you."

"It was my fault."

"Do you think you can stand?" I wanted to get her into the ambulance and out of the turmoil.

"Maybe." On shaky legs, with Eileen on one side and me on the other, Missy made her way to the ambulance and sat on the crew seat, leaving room for others who might need the stretcher. To relieve her anxiety, I would have preferred to transport her alone in her own ambulance, but I couldn't. We were down to two rigs from our usual three and didn't want to take both out of service unless we absolutely had to.

"I'm going to give you something to help your breathing," I said. We didn't carry paper bags, which were the treatment of choice for hyperventilation, but we had the next best thing. I unwrapped a non-rebreather face mask, pulled the rubber gasket from one of the side ports, and handed it to her. The small holes would allow limited fresh air to enter the mask, so she would be breathing primarily her own exhaled air. I had used this technique before and it had always broken the cycle of hyperventilation.

"I want you to hold this and keep it over your face. Breathe in and out as slowly as you can. Keep thinking about slowing your breathing down."

As I fastened Missy's seat belt and listened to her breathing ease, Jack and Stephanie arrived with a young man on the stretcher and a fully ambulatory, seemingly uninjured girl. The girl climbed into the rig and sat on the crew bench. Jack and Stephanie lifted the stretcher into position and I heard the mechanism lock it into place.

"Jen," Missy screamed. "Are you hurt?"

"I'm fine, Missy. And so's Mitch. He's got a bump on his knee but that's about it."

"But it's my fault," Missy shrieked, again panting.

"It is not," Mitch said. "I just lost it. It's no one's fault."

"But—"

"And everyone's fine," I said. "You're fine, and your friends are fine. See?"

"I don't feel well," Missy said. She paused. "I can't feel my fingers at all."

"I'm sure you can't," I said. "You've got to slow your breathing."

"Yeah, Missy," the boy said. "Just be cool. We're fine."

"But it's my fault."

"Why is it your fault?" I asked. "You were a passenger."

The boy spoke up. "She saw a bug on my collar

and went to bat it off. I turned to look at her and just lost control."

Missy's breathing was speeding up again. "See? My fault."

"Missy, relax," the girl on the stretcher said. "We're fine."

Missy looked at her friend. "You're . . . bleeding."

"It's just a cut lip," Jen said. "Chill out."

"I don't feel well," Missy said. "I'm going to faint and I've got pains in my chest."

"Of course you do," I said. "It's from all that fast breathing."

"Can I lie down?"

Stephanie had finished taking Jen's vitals and was now wrapping a BP cuff around Mitch's upper arm. The two of them slid down the crew bench and Missy stretched out on it. We strapped her down, seat-belted everyone else, and Sam began the trip to FGH. Missy lay with her eyes closed and I talked to Jen and Mitch while Stephanie started two PCRs, one for each of her patients. I had all of Missy's information and I'd do my PCR at the hospital.

As we ignored Missy, her breathing slowed. Suddenly she said, "I'm so sorry," and her breathing began to speed up again. Each time the conversation moved to the other two young people and Missy wasn't in the center of things, she moaned, her breathing quickened, and she added another complaint about her condition.

By the time we arrived at the hospital, she was suffering from chest pains, general weakness, numbness in her arms and legs, and a severe headache. We took Jen and Mitch into the ER, then put the stretcher back into the rig, moved Missy onto it, and wheeled her into her own cubicle.

I gave a report to Patty Stewart, a young ER nurse. "I think this is all hyperventilation. Every time we seemed to be ignoring her, it got worse." I listed all her complaints. "I suggest she be put somewhere away from the other two. They seem to make her anxiety worse."

Patty grinned. "Already done."

A while later, when we were ready to leave, I stuck my head into Missy's cubicle. She was lying quite comfortably with a paper bag over her face. "Feel good, Missy," I said.

"Oh, I will," she said, beaming.

God, I love teenagers.

And sometimes adults aren't much better.

Jack Jamison had been born weighing slightly under five pounds. It was the last time in his life that anyone thought of him as small. By the time he was in third grade he towered over his classmates and outweighed any two of the girls. It wasn't that Jack was fat, he was simply huge. As he grew older, he grew larger. In high school he was recruited by the football coach, but despite his size, he wasn't an asset to the team. A bit clumsy and decidedly nonconfrontational, he eventually dropped football and concentrated on his studies.

When he graduated, there was no thought of college. He worked at his father's gas station and blended in as well as a huge man could. In his early twenties he met Adele, a woman as tiny as he was huge, and eventually they married and had four children.

As the years progressed, Jack began to have medical problems, in part due to his size and increasing weight. He developed diabetes. His circulation slowed and his heart labored. His legs swelled and soon he was having difficulty walking. In his fifties, he was forced to accept his limitations, so he sold the gas station his father had left him and lived off state disability, the money from the sale, and his wife's small income from her job at a beauty salon.

At the age of sixty-one, he weighed over four hundred pounds. He told himself that his weight was under control, but his grossly swollen ankles told a different story. He spent almost all of his time in a large lounge chair, and when he moved he was slow and hesitant. Finally he needed a walker to get around. He left the house only to visit his doctor, and every day he tried to remember which of his medications to take and when to take them. Between the medications for his diabetes, his high blood pressure, and his recent bout of flu, he liked to kid that after he took his morning pills, if he shook his belly he would sound like a pair of maracas.

One morning he got out of bed, shuffled to the bathroom, took his medications, and emptied his bladder. As he shuffled toward the door to let the dog out, the exuberant German shepherd galloped beneath Jack's feet. Unable to move quickly enough to avoid the eighty-pound animal, Jack tumbled over it and landed in a heap on the floor. "Adele!" he bellowed. "Help me."

Adele rushed in from the kitchen, where she had been preparing breakfast, and, seeing Jack on the floor, began to laugh. "I've fallen and I can't get up," she said through her giggles.

"Don't be a fool, woman," Jack said. "I fell onto the

edge of the coffee table and I think I've broken a few ribs."

Sobering instantly, she hustled to Jack's side. "Oh, baby, I'm so sorry. Does it hurt really badly?"

"Of course it does," he snapped. "And I can't get my breath."

"Do you think you can make it to your chair?"

Catching his breath slowly, Jack began to maneuver his enormous frame into a sitting position. After about five minutes of grabbing and pulling, shifting and grunting, and considerable pain, he managed to get himself into his lounge chair. Now covered with sweat, he said, "This hurts like holy hell."

"You hit your head too," Adele said, getting a towel from the bathroom and patting a very sore spot on Jack's scalp. As she removed the towel she gasped. "There's a lot of blood," she said, showing her husband the red-splotched towel.

"And my ribs hurt something awful. Maybe you'd better get me an ambulance."

The pagers went off. "Fairfax Police to all home units. An EMT and an attendant are needed for a man who fell at 126 Jackson Lane. Any available unit, please call in."

I had just finished checking my e-mail and had some time available, so I called in. "Jackson Lane is in that old section behind the old railroad station, isn't it?" I asked Mark Thomas, the police dispatcher.

"Yes, Joan. It's the second left off of Hamilton."

"Okay," I said. "Tell them I'll meet the rig at the scene."

I put the green light on the top of my car and drove toward Jackson Lane. That section of town was filled with forty- and fifty-year-old houses, many of which had begun their life as summer homes and had later been converted for year-round use. After a few wrong turns, I arrived at 126 Jackson Lane, to be met by Police Officer Will McAndrews.

"Hi, Joan," he said. "This is going to be a tough one. This guy must go four hundred pounds easy."

"Shit," I muttered. "We'll need lots of lifting help."

"I already called for the fire department."

Crash kit in hand, I walked up the narrow path to the front door, opened the door, and called, "Ambulance!"

"Down here," a woman's voice called.

Goody, I thought. Down a flight of stairs. If he was as big as Will had said, this was going to be a really tough call. I made my way through the house and down the narrow stairs to the rec room. As I caught sight of my patient, I took a deep breath. "Hello, sir," I said. It was obvious that Will hadn't underestimated. "What happened to you this morning?"

"I tripped . . . over . . . the goddamn . . . dog," he said.

"What hurts?" I asked, taking in the blood-soaked towel and the man's puffing.

"My ribs. It hurts . . . when I breathe . . . deep."

"Okay, just hold still for me. How about your head?"

"He must have caught it on the corner of the coffee table," a tiny woman who stood beside the mammoth man said. She was as tall standing as he was sitting.

"My name's Joan," I said.

"I'm Adele Jamison," the woman said, "and that's my husband, Jack."

"Okay," I said, totally overwhelmed by the enormity of my task. "Are you dizzy? Did you lose consciousness when you fell?"

"No," Jack said, his breathing shallow and a bit fast.

"Any neck or back pain?"

"No," he said.

My mind whirled. If we had to immobilize him, with a collar and such, our long backboard would never hold his weight, and his body would hang off all four sides. Even our stretcher had a weight limit of 350 pounds. I slipped on a pair of gloves and palpated Jack's head, neck, and back. No pain or deformity, no point tenderness, and just a tiny amount of swelling. So far so good. I held up three fingers. "How many fingers?" I asked.

With a wicked grin, Jack said, "Five, but two of them . . . are tucked under."

I smiled. "I see your sense of humor is not too badly damaged."

"Oh, he's always like that," his wife said. "Such a kidder." She beamed at him.

"How's the head?" I asked Jack.

"Okay," he said. "Scared Adele . . . to death though . . . but it looks worse . . . than it is."

"Well, that's great," I said, "since we're going to have enough trouble getting you out of here without any added complications." I felt his ribs and found the site of his pain. I couldn't feel anything specifically broken, but I certainly couldn't rule it out.

As I reached over to take his pulse, I heard the ambulance pull up in front of the house. I keyed my radio. "45–24 to duty rig."

"45–01 on." I recognized Steve Nesbitt's voice.

"Bring in a large BP cuff and some O_2. We're going to need to discuss this one before we transport."

"10–4, Joan."

I quickly ascertained that Jack's pulse was 88, and his

shallow respirations were 24 a minute, both a bit high but still well within normal limits.

When Steve arrived at the foot of the stairs, I saw his eyes widen. "Has someone called for extra help?" he asked.

"Fire department's on the way," Will, who had followed Steve down the stairs, said.

"Great," Steve said.

I grabbed the large BP cuff and took Jack's blood pressure. Surprisingly, it was only 125 over 82, quite low for a man of his size. I gave him the numbers.

"Yeah," he said. "I'm on a strong water pill and that seems to take care of it."

"Is there another way in or out of here?" Steve asked.

"We've got a garage," Adele said.

"Let me see it," Steve said, handing me the oxygen.

As I started to place the oxygen mask over Jack's face, he pushed it away. "Later. Not now. I gotta go."

"But you need this to help you breathe."

"In a few minutes," he said, glaring at the mask. "I gotta go."

Now wanting to make an issue just yet, I said, "Okay for now. Jack, you may have noticed that you're a big guy. You will probably need a few stitches on that head injury and you might have a few broken ribs. It's going to take some doing to get you out of here."

"I can walk," he said, putting one hand on his walker.

"Nope," I said. "We need to protect your body from additional injury."

Jack raised one eyebrow. "I'm gonna walk right now 'cause I gotta pee, lady. Damn water pills."

"Let us get you a urinal," I said. "I don't want you walking around."

"Not a chance, lady," Jack said. "I don't pee into any bottle." With much grunting and heaving, he got to a standing position.

"But, sir—" I said.

"I don't think you can stop me," he said, maneuvering his walker into position. While I watched, helpless to stop him but glad he could move around by himself, he shuffled toward the bathroom, grunting with every step. "Adele," he said at the bathroom door, "help me with my pants."

As Adele hustled into the bathroom, Steve returned with three Fairfax firefighters. "We're clearing a path through the garage," he said. "It's not great but at least we won't have to climb the stairs." Phil Ortiz, our third crew member, came in through the garage door, pulling the stretcher.

"Wonderful," I said, counting the number of hands we'd have to lift our patient.

"I understand he's a big guy," Phil said.

"You said a mouthful," Steve said. He looked at the empty chair. "Where is he?"

"In the john," I said. "I couldn't stop him."

"How big is he?" one of the firefighters asked.

"Big," I said as the bathroom door opened and Jack appeared, followed by his wife.

"Oh, Jesus," I heard someone hiss.

I indicated the stretcher, raised to a height of about three feet off the ground. "We can't have him on this while it's up this high," I said. "It will never hold the weight and it'll be terribly top-heavy." Steve and Phil lowered the stretcher to its lowest position, only about fifteen inches off the ground.

"Sir," Steve said, "do you think you can sit down on here if we all help you?"

"If you put the back up all the way. I can't lie down."

Steve lifted the back of the stretcher until it was positioned so that the patient would be sitting bolt upright. "How's this?"

Using his walker to assist him, Jack shuffled toward the stretcher. With Steve on one side, one of the firefighters on the other, and Phil and another firefighter behind to support him, Jack slowly sat on the stretcher. As his full weight landed I heard protests from the metal bars, but the stretcher held. What we would have done if Jack hadn't been able to walk I didn't even want to consider. I quickly strapped him down, amazed that the stretcher seat-belt straps fit over his girth. His feet stuck off the bottom by about six inches and his head cleared the top of the back.

Steve and Phil pulled while Will and I guided the back end toward the garage. With some grunting and quiet swearing, the group of us got Jack over the sill, through the garage, and out to the rig. Three men on either side and Will at the foot lifted the stretcher into the rig. Phil and I guided it into place and listened as it locked into the mechanism on the floor of the rig. "Can any of you follow us to the hospital?" I asked. Their presence would make things much easier. We could call for extra lifting help at FGH, but locating enough manpower to lift Jack and the stretcher from the back of the ambulance would take several minutes.

"Sure," one of the firefighters said. He looked at his buddies. "Let's take my car, then I'll drop you back here afterward."

Three others nodded.

Jack allowed me to put him on oxygen in the ambulance, and, after a short drive, we arrived at FGH. As we switched him to a portable oxygen cylinder and opened the back door, I saw the car with the firefighters pull into the parking area. Again, with lots of noise and heavy breathing, they lifted Jack from the ambulance and set the stretcher onto the ground. "Don't raise it," Steve said. "I don't think it will take the strain."

We wheeled Jack into the emergency department. Rosemary Harper, one of the ER nurses on duty that morning, just stared. In the cubicle, we had to raise the stretcher to get it even with the hospital gurney, even in the gurney's lowest position. The eight of us lifted and held onto the stretcher while Jack skootched onto the gurney.

"I hope this can take the weight," I said to Rosemary.

"I think it will hold," she said. "What's his story?"

"He fell over his dog," I said. "He denies loss of consciousness, dizziness, and shows no sign of serious head injury. He's got a small, open laceration to the top of his head, and the bleeding was controlled before my arrival. He's got possible broken ribs on the right side." I pointed to the location of Jack's rib injury.

"Can't I sit in a chair?" Jack asked.

"No," Rosemary said. "We'll have to get you to X ray, and that means wheeling you around. Just be patient with us for a few minutes."

We removed the oxygen mask from Jack's face and Rosemary replaced it with a nasal canula, which would satisfy his body's need for a little extra oxygen. As I completed my paperwork, I saw Adele hustle in from the admitting area. "Is he okay?" she asked.

"He's doing fine," I answered.

"That's good," she said. "Where is he?" We then heard a voice yell, "Someone get me to the bathroom. I've got to pee again."

Adele sighed. "Those new water pills make us both crazy."

I found out later that he was treated and released. His ribs were badly bruised but not broken. Ed and I spent quite a while thinking through what we would have done if Jack's injuries had been more serious. "Take out a wall," Ed said, only slightly facetiously, "and get a forklift."

Hank Morgan liked to drink. He didn't consider himself an alcoholic since he could go days or even a week without any alcohol. But he liked his whiskey. Boilermakers were his drink of choice, and most Friday evenings you would find him at the Red Foxx Lounge with his buddies, tossing back boilermakers and watching whatever sports were in season.

It was basketball playoffs and again the Chicago Bulls were trampling their West Coast rivals. Michael Jordan made sensational play after sensational play, which frequently were celebrated with another round of drinks. Hank had driven to the bar with his friend Joe because Joe managed to enjoy their evenings out without any booze. As designated driver, when the game was over and the celebrating done, he drove several of the guys home, including Hank.

Hank arrived home at almost one, feeling very good. The Bulls had beaten the spread and he was twenty bucks richer. As usual, by the time he arrived home, his wife, Doris, and his three kids were already asleep. As also often happened, he was very sick to his stomach. He dumped his light jacket on the chair and headed for the bathroom. Without even turning on the light, he stumbled to the bowl, leaned over, and threw up with such force that it caused a sharp pain to knife from his breastbone to his spine. Piss, he thought. I must have thrown my damn back out.

He fumbled his way to his bed and dropped on it, in too much pain to worry about removing his clothes. He lay still for a while and, although the pain lessened only a small amount, he fell into a half sleep, half stupor. A few hours later he awoke feeling terrible. He was weak, breathless, and the pain was intense. He was also very sick to his stomach and very thirsty. Probably from the booze, he reasoned. Trying not to wake his wife and have to listen to her lecture on the evils of drinking, he staggered to the bathroom in the dark, threw up again, and drank two full glasses of water.

Back in bed, he found he was unable to sleep. He lingered for an hour somewhere between sleep and wakefulness, then again staggered to the bathroom. This time he felt so weak that he had to hold on to the bed table, the doorknob, and the counter to make it. As he grabbed for the bowl, he knocked over the bathroom glass and it fell to the tile with a loud crash.

"You okay?" Doris mumbled as the crash awakened her.

"I don't know," Hank said weakly.

At the strange sound of her husband's voice, Doris climbed out of bed, walked quickly to the bathroom door, and flipped on the light. The floor was covered with blood. "Baby," she said. "Where did you cut yourself? You're bleeding everywhere."

Hank turned his head from the bowl and looked at the

floor. "I don't know," he said. "I don't think I cut myself at all." He glanced at the water in the toilet and almost passed out. The water in the bowl was bright red. "Oh my God," he said.

Doris took one look into the toilet and ran to call 911.

Ed and I were riding the midnight to 6 A.M. shift that morning. We usually rode only Sunday nights, but Heather and Tom Franks, originally signed up for the shift, had called earlier that afternoon. Tom's mother had become ill and they asked whether we could fill in for them. "No problem," I had said.

"It's usually quiet anyway," Tom had answered. "We haven't gone out in over two months."

"Thanks," I said acidly. "You've probably jinxed it now."

When the phone awakened me from a deep sleep about 3:30 A.M. I flashed on Tom's words. "What's up?" I said into the phone.

"It's Bob," the voice said. "We've got a call at 87 Hill-crest for a man bleeding. I'm at headquarters so I'll bring the rig."

"Okay. We'll meet you at the scene."

Ed was already partly dressed. "That was Bob Fiorella." As I dressed I told him about the call, and in only a few moments we were speeding toward Hillcrest. During the drive we were silent, each trying to gather our thoughts. The abrupt transition from sleep to action is a difficult one, but after ten years of riding nights, both Ed and I have become accustomed to it. It's been said that you can get used to anything.

We arrived at almost the same moment as the ambulance. As Ed and Bob got the trauma bag and oxygen from the rig, I sprinted up the front walk and knocked on the door. Police Officer Merve Berkowitz opened it and, speechless, pointed to the end of the hall.

"Hello," I called as I walked down the carpeted hallway to the master bedroom. "Fairfax Ambulance."

"In here," a woman's voice called.

I entered the bedroom and saw three boys who appeared to be between the ages of ten and fifteen, all clustered at the bathroom door. They backed away, forming a path for me. I stepped into the bathroom to be greeted by the unmistakable smell of fresh blood. I instinctively moved my tongue around the inside of my mouth, tasting the metallic smell. The floor was covered with it, combined with shards of broken glass. A man was sitting on the floor, leaning on the closed lid of the toilet.

"Where are you cut?" I asked.

"I don't think he's cut at all." The woman was tucked in a corner of the small room, dustpan and brush in hand. "I'm trying to clean up the glass. But I think he's vomiting the blood."

"Don't flush," I said as the man's hand reached to empty the bowl. I tiptoed gingerly around the glass and, moving the man aside, lifted the lid. The water was bright red. I know as well as anyone that a small amount of blood mixed into water usually looks just as bright as the undiluted blood would look, but the intensity of the color impressed me.

"Sir," I asked, "when did this start?"

"When I got home last evening," he said weakly. "I threw up and I think my back went out. Hurts real bad here"—he pointed to his chest—"right through to the back."

"Did you throw up blood then?"

"I don't know. I didn't turn the light on."

"What time was that?" I asked, leaning down to grab his wrist.

"About one. Maybe one-thirty."

I reflexively glanced at my watch. It was now after three-thirty. I found the man's pulse but it was weak and thready. His face was deathly pale and damp from sweat, and his breathing was rapid. Behind me, the woman was sweeping up glass. "Where did the glass come from?" I asked.

She looked up. "It must have broken when he came into the bathroom. I thought he had cut himself but when I saw the blood in the john, I called you."

"You did the right thing. I'm Joan."

"I'm Doris," the woman said, "and this is my husband, Henry."

"Hank," the man said weakly.

"Okay, Hank. We're going to get you to the hospital and let them check you out."

He just nodded. Ed, Merve, and Bob helped me get Hank out of the bathroom and onto the stretcher. "Let's put him in the Trendelenburg position," I said.

"Right," Ed said, quickly adjusting the back of the stretcher flat and raising the foot to elevate Hank's legs and help his circulation. Bob pulled the pillow from beneath Hank's head and put him on oxygen. We quickly took a set of vitals, all of which indicated that he was already in shock and his body was having severe trouble coping with the loss of blood.

As Ed and Bob strapped Hank onto the stretcher, I tried to get as much information from Doris as I could. "Where was he before this happened?"

"He went drinking with a few friends. He usually gets

home late, so the boys and I went to bed. He must have come in after one, but he didn't wake me. You should have awakened me," she said to her husband.

He closed his eyes and didn't answer.

When we were ready to move, I glanced again at my watch. We had been on the scene for eleven minutes. Not bad. In cases like this, ten minutes on the scene was ideal.

In EMS we have lots of "sayings." The "golden hour" is one. It's our aim to get a seriously injured or ill patient from his home through the emergency room and to the operating room in under an hour. To do this we "scoop and run" on occasion, moving as quickly as we can to the ER. When we don't have a seriously ill or injured patient, we have time to "stay and play."

We scooped and ran with Hank. With Mrs. Morgan in the front with Bob, we sped through the deserted town to FGH.

In the emergency room, while a nurse started an IV line, Dr. Morrison quickly evaluated our patient. He ordered chest X rays and, as I finished the paperwork, he called Mrs. Morgan into a small side cubicle. "Does your husband drink a lot?" I heard him ask.

"Most Fridays he goes out drinking with his friends. Why?"

"I think your husband has a ruptured esophagus. It happens occasionally with heavy drinkers."

"He's not an alcoholic. He likes to drink some, but he can do without it when he needs to. Is this serious?"

"It can be. We don't have all the tests back yet, but he's a pretty sick guy. We've got a surgeon on the way and unless I'm very much mistaken, your husband will be in the OR within the hour."

We were done with our paperwork and I stepped into the small area. "Mrs. Morgan, I hope everything goes all right with your husband."

"Thank you so much," she said. "You got there so fast."

"I'm glad we could help."

Several months later I ran into Mrs. Morgan in the supermarket. She pulled her cart into line behind me and stared for a minute. "Aren't you with the ambulance?" she asked.

"Yes."

"I'm Doris Morgan. You probably don't remember but you picked my husband up about three months ago."

"I certainly do remember," I said, worrying that she was going to tell me something I didn't want to hear. The man had been near death when we last saw each other.

"He's out of the hospital and doing okay," she said.

Relieved, I smiled. "I'm so glad. How did it go after I left you in the emergency room?"

"They told me he had probably ruptured his food pipe when he first threw up. His chest cavity filled with blood and with the water he was drinking because he was so thirsty. He had one and then two collapsed lungs."

"Wow," I said.

"The thoracic surgeon wouldn't operate so they heli-coptered him to the trauma center. They operated that day and he was so sick for a long time. He had a bad infection and ran a fever of 103. He was in the hospital for eight weeks. I remember he went in on a Saturday and came home on a Saturday."

"How are you holding up?"

"I'm okay. I'm tough and so are my kids. My oldest

wouldn't go to the hospital after the first time and I couldn't blame him. The other two went with me alternate days. We all actually thought he wouldn't make it. But he did."

"And he's fine now?"

"Pretty much. No smoking, no drinking, but other that that, he's good."

I finished unloading my groceries on the belt and watched the checker scanning my items from the corner of my eye. "I'm delighted that everything turned out well," I said.

"Me too. And thanks again for getting there so quickly."

"You're very welcome. And I'm glad you called so fast."

"The doctor said that if we'd waited another hour, he might not have made it."

I handed the checker enough money to pay for my groceries and loaded the bags into my cart. "Please remember me to your husband," I said.

"I will. And thanks again."

Chapter 4

Michael and Claire O'Hearn had been my neighbors for twenty-five years. We had lived in parallel worlds that never quite touched. Our houses were directly across the street from each other, but we raised our children on our side of the street and they raised their children on their side. We would exchange an occasional "Hi, Michael," "Hi, Ed" as I would pull into or out of my driveway. I would wave at their children and they would wave back. Their sons seemed to spend all of their waking hours shooting hoops in their driveway while my daughters liked to play indoors.

I would have short conversations with Claire or Michael when we met at the mailboxes, and I often thought that I'd like to get to know them better. But the years raced by, the children grew up, and it never happened. After Michael retired from his job as a police officer, we sometimes chatted while taking a break from shoveling snow from our driveways. But there was never any more interaction than that.

It was the evening of St. Patrick's Day. I was working late in my basement office. The TV news was on—filled with the usual banalities about everyone being Irish on

St. Patrick's Day. Suddenly the house began to vibrate. Puzzled, I walked upstairs and heard the sounds of bagpipes coming from outside. I opened the front door, peered out, and was enveloped by the magnificent drone and cry of bagpipes and the rattle of drums. It took me a while to realize that the music was not coming from a radio that had its volume turned up. As my eyes adjusted to the dark, I could see figures on Michael and Claire's lawn, silhouetted against the light of the porch.

I threw on my jacket and walked down my driveway. A small crowd was collecting in front of the O'Hearn house as neighbors were drawn to the sound of the pipes. Michael sat on the porch, bundled up against the March cold, surrounded by his family. Claire stood next to him, her hand on his shoulder. On the lawn, facing Michael, stood the tall, shadowy figures of at least twenty-five men in traditional Irish formal military dress, playing bagpipes and drums. My neighbor Harve came up beside me.

"Michael's dying, you know," he said.

"No." I gasped. "I knew he had been ill, but I didn't know it was that bad."

"They've given him only a very short time," Harve said.

We were silent for the next fifteen or twenty minutes as the majestic sound of pipes and drums swirled through our suburban neighborhood on that dark St. Patrick's Day night. After the music stopped, the pipers walked, single file, up to the porch and greeted Michael, who smiled and spoke to each of them. I saw a number of the pipers wipe their eyes as they walked past me.

I had been back in my house for about two hours when my pager began to beep. "GVK–861 Prescott Fire to the rescue squad. Be advised the ambulance is responding with a full crew for a possible DOA." He gave the address. It was the O'Hearn house.

I threw on my jacket and ran down my driveway and across the street. I rang the bell and Claire opened the door. "Oh, Ed. I think he's gone." I walked over to the sofa where Michael's wasted body lay. He seemed to be asleep, but he was not breathing and his skin was gray. I knelt and pressed my fingers against the side of his neck. There was no pulse. I turned to Claire. "I'm so sorry," I said.

"Please don't try to do anything for him," Claire said. "He didn't want anything done."

"Do you have a DNR?" I asked, hoping that the do-not-resuscitate order would be in a form I could accept.

"No, but I have a health care proxy."

I felt a moment of panic. Without being shown a signed DNR order, I would be required to begin CPR, which the responding ambulance crew would continue during transport. Maybe this was an "obvious" death. I lifted Michael's arm and looked at the skin that had been resting on the sofa. It was purple—dependent lividity—a criterion of obvious death. Relieved, I stood up and turned to Michael's family. "He must have died right after the pipers were here," I said. "It's okay. I'll talk to the ambulance crew. I'll make sure they don't do anything."

That night I lay awake for hours thinking about the awesome physical and emotional responsibilities of being an EMT, about two families separated by a narrow street, and about how joyful Michael must have felt to be escorted out of this life by loving family and friends to the ancient sounds of pipes and drums.

* * *

I sometimes become impatient when working with old-time paramedics who never seem to get excited, no matter how urgent the situation. Although I am fully aware of the need to remain calm under pressure, I find it difficult not to yell "Hurry up, damn it" when I'm doing CPR on a patient in cardiac arrest while the paramedic, calm to the point of seeming on the verge of nodding off, slowly turns on his defibrillator, checks the patient's heart rhythm, and prepares to administer a shock that will, it is hoped, "restart" the patient's heart.

But it is more dangerous when an emergency care-giver overreacts to a situation. An inexperienced EMT may confuse anxiety-induced hyperventilation with a heart attack or a minor but bloody scalp laceration with a serious head injury and, in doing so, may make the situation more difficult. Sometimes, however, at the scene of a highly stressful emergency medical situation, even an experienced paramedic or EMT may panic and a newly arrived caregiver may be able to provide a calmer and more appropriate approach to the situation.

It was a cold, crystal-clear February morning in Fairfax. A thin coating of fresh snow covered the seven or eight inches that had accumulated during the previous week. I had just taken my cross-country skis, poles, and boots out of the closet and was getting ready to head toward the Redtail Ridge golf course—one of Fairfax's best places for cross-country skiing—when my pager went off.

"GBY–639 Fairfax Police to all FVAC pagers and home monitors. A full crew is needed for a child who fell on the ice in front of 2123 Willow Valley Road. Please call in."

I leaned my skis against the wall, careful not to get any fiberglass splinters in my fingers, which I often did when handling them without gloves. The skis were the expensive no-wax kind, but touching them was like handling a pair of fine-quilled porcupines. I picked up the phone and dialed Fairfax Police.

"Fairfax Police, Dispatcher Thomas speaking."

"Hi, Mark. It's Ed Herman. I'll go directly to the scene. Get an attendant and a driver to pick up the rig."

"Okay, Ed. You'd better get there stat. I have an officer on the scene who thinks the boy is very badly hurt. He seems to be paralyzed."

Oh shit, I thought. The address on Willow Valley Road, a main road between Fairfax and Prescott, was about halfway between my house and FVAC headquarters. I would be the first medical responder on the scene and I would be in charge. I knew that with a back or neck injury, the slightest movement could cause permanent paralysis or death. If the accident had happened in Prescott, a paramedic would have responded and would have been in charge, but, since Fairfax did not yet have paramedic service, it would be up to me, as the first EMT on the scene.

"I'm on my way, Mark," I said.

I dashed to my car, quickly brushed the snow off the back window and windshield, switched on my green light, and headed for Willow Valley Road.

As I approached the scene, I could see Officer Chuck Harding kneeling over someone who lay on the driveway in front of a brown-and-white Tudor-style house. I pulled

over, jumped out of my car, and almost fell flat on my
face as my shoes slid on the thin layer of ice. A group of
bystanders parted as I skated toward them. A boy in his
early teens lay faceup on the pavement. Chuck was
holding the boy's head between his hands to keep it from
moving.

"What have you got, Chuck?" I asked, kneeling next
to him.

Chuck's voice was tight and guarded. "His legs are
paralyzed and he can't feel anything in his feet."

I could feel my own throat tense as I turned to the boy
and pretended to be calm. "Hi, my name's Ed. What's
yours?"

"It's Jason," a woman's voice yelled from behind me.
"Jason Gottlieb."

I looked up at a fortyish-looking woman who appeared
wide-eyed. "Are you his mother?" I asked.

"Yes," the woman replied. "I'm Marion Gottlieb."

"Mrs. Gottlieb, I need to have Jason answer himself.
Okay?"

"Yeah, sure. All right."

I turned back to the boy. "How old are you, Jason?"

"I'm fourteen," he said, his teeth chattering.

"Jason, can you tell me what happened?"

"I was running and I slipped on the ice. I fell on my
back."

"What is hurting you now?"

"My back. It hurts real bad, especially when I try to
move."

"Well, I don't want you to move. I want you to be as
still as you can while I examine you. Officer Harding is
holding your head to keep it from moving. When I ask

you questions, I want you to answer yes or no but don't nod or shake your head. Okay?"

"Yeah," the boy answered. He was obviously frightened and in a lot of pain but was trying to act brave.

With Jason lying on his back and the heavy winter clothing that he was wearing, it was going to be impossible to palpate his spine for point tenderness or deformity. "Does anything hurt other than your back?" I asked.

"No," Jason whimpered, "but my back hurts so much."

"Jason, can you move your hands?" I asked.

The boy lifted his arms and wiggled his fingers. I placed the index and middle fingers of each of my hands in his palms. "I want you to squeeze my fingers as hard as you can with both hands," I said.

Jason squeezed my fingers weakly.

I moved down to his feet and pressed my thumb down on the toe of his winter boot. "Can you feel me touching you?" I asked.

"No," Jason replied.

"Can you move your feet?" I asked.

"No."

"Jason, I want you to move your feet," I ordered sternly. Nothing happened.

"Oh, no. Oh, God!" Jason's mother cried.

I turned to Chuck. "I'll take over head stabilization. Radio police headquarters and ask them to see whether Dr. O'Grady's available to come over. I'd rather not move this boy until he is evaluated by a doctor."

Chuck released Jason's head, stood up, and spoke into his portable radio.

I felt that I was in way over my head. We had to get Jason to the hospital, but if his spine had been fractured, as seemed likely, the slightest movement could result in permanent paralysis. I was panic stricken and desperately wanted to avoid the responsibility for any action that could have such disastrous consequences. Although we had no paramedics in Fairfax, Dr. O'Grady, one of the local physicians, was an emergency medicine specialist and was willing to respond to the scene of critical situations when he was available.

After he finished his radio traffic, Chuck knelt at Jason's head and resumed manual stabilization. "Our dispatcher will try to get Dr. O'Grady," he said.

I heard the wail of a siren as the FVAC ambulance pulled up. Pam Kovacs and Jack McCaffrey strode over. "What do you need, Ed?" Pam asked.

"Just a regular C-collar right now," I said. "I've asked for Dr. O'Grady, if he's available."

"What do you have?" Jack asked as Pam went to the ambulance for a cervical collar.

"A fourteen-year-old boy with a possible spinal fracture," I answered.

Pam returned with the collar and, with Chuck still holding stabilization, she placed it around Jason's neck.

"I'll get the longboard, spider straps, and head blocks," Pam said, turning toward the rig.

"Okay," I said. "But I don't want to do anything until Dr. O'Grady gets here. I want the boy to be evaluated before we try to move him."

Pam stopped and turned back to me. "Can I speak to you for a minute, Ed?" she asked.

"Sure, Pam. Jack, would you stay with Jason?"

"Okay, Ed," Jack replied, taking my place at Jason's side.

I walked a few steps to where Pam was standing. "What's up, Pam?" I asked.

"Ed, you were first on the scene so you're the EMT in charge, but do you really think it's a good idea to wait for Dr. O'Grady before we immobilize the boy and get him out of the cold? He's shivering pretty badly and we may soon have to deal with hypothermia as well as a possible spinal fracture."

"I know you're right, Pam. But I'm afraid to move him before Dr. O'Grady gets here."

"Ed. What difference will Dr. O'Grady make? We're far more experienced at doing spinal immobilization than he is. No matter what he finds, we still have to do what we're trained to do."

I looked at Pam and suddenly realized that she was right. The fact that Dr. O'Grady had much more medical knowledge than we had made no difference. Pam, Jack, and I knew as much about how to do a spinal immobilization as he did, and we were more experienced. The responsibility was ours and since I was crew chief, it was, in the final analysis, mine. I nodded. "You're right, Pam. Let's do what we have to do," I said, then turned toward Jack. "Jack. You and Pam get the immobilization equipment."

I walked over to Jason's mother. "We're going to immobilize Jason on a board and get him into the ambulance to warm him up. If Dr. O'Grady gets here before we're ready to leave, fine, but we're not going to delay transportation to wait for him."

"All right," the woman replied. "You do whatever you think best."

I kneeled next to Jason, as Officer Harding continued to hold head stabilization. "How are you doing, Jason?" I asked.

"My back hurts a lot and I'm real cold," he said through chattering teeth.

"We're going to get you into a warm ambulance. But first we have to put you on a board to protect your neck and back while we move you. We'll have to truss you up like a turkey, even though Thanksgiving is over. Yes?"

"Yes," Jason replied with a small smile.

"Listen, Jason. I don't think there's any way that we can move you without it hurting, but we'll be as gentle as possible."

"It's all right," Jason whimpered.

Pam and Jack arrived with the longboard, spider straps, and head blocks. "How do you want to do it, Ed? Logroll?"

I looked at Jason. In examining him, the slightest movement had caused him to cry out in pain. Logrolling him onto a backboard would be horrendous.

"No. Let's use the scoop," I said. "That can get him onto the longboard with the least movement."

Although the metal scissorslike scoop stretcher would not provide enough spinal immobilization for transporting Jason, it would enable us to lift him onto a board without the need to roll him onto his side.

Pam and Jack quickly returned with the two separate pieces of the scoop stretcher. Placing them on either side of Jason, they adjusted the sides to the proper length to fit the boy's body. Then, while Officer Harding lifted Jason's head slightly, continuing to maintain head stabilization, the two upper ends of the scoop were slid under his head and shoulders and snapped into place. Then, at Jason's feet, I began to pull the lower ends of the scoop toward each other. The ends were almost together but I was unable to lock them so that we could lift the boy.

Feeling under Jason's body, I found that the right side of the scoop was caught under his buttock. "We're going to have to roll him to the left just a little," I said.

Pam and Jack got into position. "On your count, Chuck," I said, knowing that control of the boy's head was of paramount importance.

Chuck began his count. "One, two, three."

As Chuck rotated Jason's head slightly to the left, Pam and Jack rolled the boy so that his head and body moved as a unit. Jason screamed with pain, but within a couple of seconds I had clicked the bottom of the scoop into place. Within a few more minutes and without any further pain, we had fully immobilized Jason on a longboard and gotten him into the ambulance.

Once in the rig, Pam and I were able to examine the boy more thoroughly. His vital signs were all normal, as were his lung sounds, and he was still shivering—which indicated that he was not seriously hypothermic. I was mostly concerned with his apparent lack of feeling in his feet and inability to move them. I carefully removed the boot from his right foot and touched his big toe. Jason's toes were icy cold but did not appear to be frostbitten. "Jason," I asked, "can you feel me touching your foot?"

"No," Jason replied.

I pinched his toe hard. "Ow," the boy yelled.

Pam and I looked at each other and we both broke into big smiles.

"Sorry, Jason. I won't do that again. But tell me which toe I pinched."

"The big one," Jason said.

"That's the right answer to the $64,000 question," Pam said, laughing.

"His toes were numb from the cold," I said to Pam. "And with those heavy boots on, we weren't able to press hard enough to get a reaction."

"Jason," I said to the boy, "can you move your toes?"

"No."

"Why not?" I asked, for the first time pursuing the question to the next level.

"My back hurts when I try to move them."

"Jason, I want you to try to move your big toe just a little bit," I said, watching the boy's foot. Jason's toe moved.

"Okay, Jason. That's great," I said with an almost overwhelming sense of relief.

I yelled to Jack, who was waiting to drive to the hospital with Mrs. Gottlieb in the passenger seat. "Okay, Jack, let's roll. Fairfax General. You can take it code 2, nice and easy. Radio Dr. O'Grady that we're transporting and he can discontinue his response." Although I had decided not to delay transportation to wait for the doctor, if my patient was unstable I might have asked him to intercept us on the way to the hospital. But Jason was doing just fine.

I leaned toward the front. "Mrs. Gottlieb," I said, loud enough for her to hear, "Jason's doing just fine. I can't tell you how seriously his back is injured, but he's not paralyzed and he does have feeling in his toes. And those are very good signs."

"Thank God," Mrs. Gottlieb whispered as we slowly began to roll toward Fairfax General Hospital.

Jason's injury turned out to be muscle and soft tissue only. His spine was not fractured and he was treated and released the same day.

*   *   *

Being a member of a fire department rescue squad has its personal advantages. If I were to have a fire or a medical emergency, the people who would respond would all be friends and acquaintances. On the other hand . . . the people who would respond would all be friends and acquaintances.

The rain had been heavy all evening, accompanied by gale-force winds. The storm was finally easing up when I noticed that bright lights were shining through my living-room window from a car in my driveway. It was late and I wasn't expecting visitors, so I went to the window to see who had arrived. My own car, with its headlights on, was the only vehicle there. I was sure that I hadn't left the headlights on, and besides, I hadn't driven the car since early that afternoon. If the headlights had been on all that time, they would have drained the battery by now. It must have been a prank by some of the neighborhood kids, I thought, although I couldn't imagine why anyone would have gone out into the storm just to turn my car headlights on.

I grabbed a flashlight and went out to my Neon. The rain had stopped but as I approached the car, I could see that I had left the driver's side window open. I looked in and saw that the floor was full of water, the front seats were soaked, and the wind had driven the rain forward so that the dashboard and even the inside of the windshield were wet. There was a strong smell of burning insulation, and wisps of smoke streamed from behind the dashboard. I opened the door, leaned in, and felt for the headlight switch. It was in the off position. Evidently, the rainwater that had run down behind the dashboard had shorted out some wires, which were now burning. Being a person who has been trained to deal with emergency situations, I acted quickly and instinctively. I ran to the house and called Joan.

"Hello," a sleepy voice answered.

"Joan, my car's on fire."

"Huh?" she replied, not very helpfully.

"I left my car windows open and the rain got in and shorted out the wires and they're burning. What should I do?"

"Call the fire department."

The thought had never occurred to me. Of course, when there's a fire you're supposed to call the fire department. How lucky I am that Joan is so smart. "That's a great idea, Joan. Thanks," I said, and hung up.

I was about to dial 911 when it hit me. Wait a minute, I thought. I *am* the fire department. If I call the fire in, I'll know all of the firefighters who respond. I imagined what would happen every time I pulled into the firehouse parking lot for the next few weeks or maybe months. "Hey, Ed, don't forget to close your car windows," or "Started any fires lately, Ed?" There was no way I could call 911. I dialed Joan's number again.

"Hello."

"I can't call the Prescott Fire Department. I'd never live it down. I'd hear about it for months. Years maybe."

"Are you crazy? If your wires are burning you have to call the fire department before the whole car goes up in flames."

"I know, I know," I replied, but there was no way that I was going to do it. Joan obviously didn't understand priorities. Better to lose the car than endure the embarrassment of calling people I knew to come to fix a mess that I had caused myself. But the car was close to the house. If it went up what about the building? I had to move the car.

I hung up the phone, ran out, jumped behind the wheel of the car, and rolled it down the driveway, almost to the street. Okay, I thought. It's far enough from the house. Now, maybe if I disconnect the battery, the wires will stop burning. Although no smoke was visible now, the car still reeked from burning plastic. I grabbed a wrench from the trunk, popped open the hood, and disconnected the battery. The headlights went out. I stood by until I was certain that no more smoke was coming from under the dashboard and the smell of burning plastic was diminishing, then, exhausted, I went to bed.

The next day I found that only the headlight switch had shorted out. None of the wiring had burned and I had no further problems after the dealer replaced the switch. And my friends in the Prescott Fire Department never knew about the fire call that they didn't get that night. Until now.

I had just dozed off. The Mets were playing on the West Coast and the game had gone into extra innings. Suddenly the bed started shaking violently and a voice shrieked "Yes. Yes."

"What? What?" I yelled, bolting upright.

"Matt Franco just hit a home run. We might win this thing after all."

With a sigh of relief I sank back into my pillow. It was neither an earthquake nor a missile attack—just the crazed sports fan that I spend a good part of my life with. I glanced at the clock. "We've been on duty for half an hour," I said. "How about turning off the TV and going to sleep?"

"I will," Joan said. "With any luck the game's almost over."

I'm a "football widower," probably one of the very few such beings that exist in the United States of America. I have no interest in spectator sports whatsoever. I have never been able to understand the concept of "rooting" for a team. Why anyone would care whether the Mets or the Bulls or the Packers win has always been a mystery to me.

Joan, on the other hand, is a sports nut. She will watch any sport and somehow will find a reason to root for one of the competing teams. I have seen her root for the Minsk Dynamos in a soccer match against the Moscow Army team. Once, while traveling in England, she spent an evening with an International Snooker Tournament on in the background for want of any other televised sport.

The game must have been over because it was dark when the telephone rang. I looked at the clock. It was 4:00 A.M.

By the time Joan hung up the phone, I was out of bed and throwing on my FVAC uniform. "What have we got?" I asked.

"A woman in labor," Joan replied. "We're going directly to the scene. The police will tone out for someone to pick up the rig."

As we dashed toward the car we could hear the police page on our portable radios. "GBY–639 to all pagers and home units. A driver is needed to pick up the ambulance for a call at 1410 Carol Road for a woman in labor. Will a driver please call in."

A call for a "woman in labor" usually means that someone wants to use the ambulance as a taxi service. At 4:00 A.M., I didn't very much appreciate being awakened in order to save someone the expense of taking a cab. But twice Joan and I had actually ended up delivering babies. The first was in the middle of an ice storm. Our patient's husband had been driving her to the hospital when his car slid off the road. No one had been injured and we began to transport the woman by ambulance, following a sand truck. When the sander got stuck on the ice, we knew we were about to deliver our first baby. Joan did the "catching" while I assisted her.

The next delivery was about a year later. This time it was on a beautiful day at the beginning of December. The baby was already crowning—the top of its head was visible—when we arrived at the scene. The woman was very concerned that her husband wasn't there. "Where is he?" Joan asked.

"He's out gathering hay," the woman replied.

Neither Joan nor I asked any further questions about the husband. We both assumed that he was planning to use the hay to cover the bottom of a manger. When Joan got into position to do the delivery, I tapped her on the shoulder. "My turn," I demanded. This time I delivered the baby and Joan suctioned its mouth and cut the umbilical cord. The woman's husband returned in time to accompany his wife and brand-new daughter to the hospital. We never learned what he did with the hay.

* * *

When we arrived at the middle-class home on a quiet suburban street, we found a twenty-one-year-old woman in what appeared to be an advanced stage of labor. From the size of her abdomen, she seemed to be in the eighth or ninth month of pregnancy. Her husband, who was sitting on the bed next to her, was very concerned.

"Hi, I'm Joan and this is Ed," Joan said.

"I'm Tim Hasbrook, and this is my wife, Gloria," the man said as his wife grimaced and squeezed his hand. Her knuckles were white with the effort.

"How long have you been in labor?" Joan asked.

"She's been having mild pains since about seven yesterday evening," the man replied, "but they suddenly started to get really bad about an hour ago. I was afraid that if I tried to drive her to the hospital, we wouldn't get there in time."

"Is this your first pregnancy, Gloria?" Joan asked.

"Yes," Gloria replied, the contraction having passed.

"When is the baby due?" Joan asked.

"It should be due pretty soon," Tim replied. "We figure that it's been about nine months since . . . You know."

"Well, what does the doctor say?"

"I haven't seen a doctor," Gloria said, grimacing with another contraction.

While Joan questioned Gloria and Tim, I checked Gloria's vital signs and timed her contractions. "Her pulse is 90, strong and regular, respirations 20, and her BP is 150 over 70," I reported. She experienced another contraction and I stared at my wristwatch while Gloria panted. "Her contractions are about 25 seconds apart and 45 seconds duration," I said.

"Can we make it to the hospital?" Tim asked.

"I think so," Joan replied. "She does seem to be pretty

well along in labor but without a doctor to examine how far her cervix is dilated, we can't be sure. First babies usually take a while. I'll take a look during the next contraction to make sure that the baby isn't crowning, and then we'll get her to the hospital."

By the time Joan had checked and made sure that the baby's head had not started to emerge, Bob Fiorella had arrived with the ambulance and had brought in the stretcher. We quickly made Gloria as comfortable as possible and within a couple of minutes were on our way to Fairfax General. Ten minutes later we transferred Gloria to a bed in "Labor and Delivery," wished her and her husband luck, and were on our way home.

A few days later, as I was about to leave the Fairfax General emergency room after bringing in the slightly injured victim of an automobile accident, Dr. Margolis spotted me. "Hey, Ed," he said. "You know that woman in labor you brought in a couple of nights ago?"

"Yeah. Did she have a boy or a girl?" I asked.

"Neither," he replied. "She wasn't pregnant. The story's all over the hospital."

In a state of near disbelief, I listened as he explained.

Tim had been asked to leave the room while an obstetric nurse examined Gloria. In a few minutes, the nurse emerged and began talking animatedly with the other nurses. About five minutes later, the resident ob-gyn went into the room. Soon after Tim was summoned into Gloria's room, where an attractive woman in her forties, with a stethoscope draped around her neck, and the nurse who had first examined Gloria stood next to his wife's bed. Gloria's eyes were closed and she appeared to be sleeping.

"I'm Dr. Mukherjee," the woman said.

Tim looked at the concerned faces of the doctor and nurse. "What's wrong?" he asked, almost panic stricken. "Is my wife all right?"

"Yes, yes," the doctor reassured him. "She's fine. I've given her something to relax her. It's just that—"

"What?" Tim demanded.

"Well, I don't know how to tell you this gently. There's no baby."

Tim looked back and forth at the discomfort evident on the faces of Dr. Mukherjee and the obstetrical nurse. Unable to comprehend, he began to look around, shouting "Don't nobody leave the room. Where's the baby? Don't nobody leave the room."

"You don't understand, Mr. Hasbrook," the doctor said. "Nobody took the baby. There never was a baby. Your wife wasn't pregnant."

"Is that really possible?" I asked Dr. Margolis, incredulous. "I saw her. She looked pregnant. I felt her abdomen tighten with contractions. She even told us how it felt when the baby kicked."

"It's called false pregnancy, or pseudopregnancy," Dr. Margolis replied. "Before we had sonograms, it occasionally fooled even doctors. It's a psychosomatic condition in which the body mimics pregnancy and even labor. Nowadays, with prenatal care, we usually detect it early, but your patient didn't have any prenatal care so she went full term with a nonexistent baby. Dr. Mukherjee put her on a diet and recommended psychological counseling."

As I left the hospital I thought to myself that, whenever an EMT thinks he's seen everything, there's something new just around the corner.

Chapter 5

At the time of the accident, Maryanne Mortolo had been a member of FVAC for eleven years and she was a good EMT. A stay-at-home mom, she had little time to devote to riding. She arranged her weeks, however, so that, except when her children needed her, she was on duty at headquarters from 6:00 A.M. to noon every Wednesday morning. She liked being helpful to the community and she loved the respect she got from her friends and relatives. And she enjoyed her weekly mornings with Rose.

Rose Weinstein had been an EMT for almost fifteen years and had ridden every Wednesday morning for all that time. Rose worked as a postal clerk in Prescott and always managed to arrange her shifts so she was free on Wednesday. That way her ambulance shifts broke up the week, and it was kind of like having two weekends. Although she went through all the skills practice and learned new techniques and protocols in her EMT refresher class, she usually let Maryanne be the one in charge, happy to drive the rig and stay in the background.

Recently Clyde Barnett had begun to ride regularly with "the ladies," as he called them. A clerk at the local Caldor's, he was relatively new to FVAC and had been an EMT for only two years. After his first morning with Maryanne and Rose, he rearranged his schedule so he could become a regular on their morning shift. He was young and eager and a good cook. So, although one of the women usually brought the makings, Clyde cooked breakfast each week.

That morning Caitlin Malloy, whom everyone called Kate, had joined them. Not yet an EMT, Kate had graduated from Fairfax High School the previous spring and was now enrolled in the local junior college, still not sure what she wanted to do with her life. Since her usual Wednesday morning class had been canceled, she had decided to make up for her lack of riding hours by signing up for this shift. And she had heard that there was usually more than enough of Clyde's good cooking.

"I love my Shakespeare class," Kate was saying, her mouth full of toast. "But what can you do with Shakespeare?"

"You should take what you enjoy," Rose said. "Soon enough you'll be stuck into something for the rest of your life. College is for tasting."

"Not necessarily," Maryanne said. "When you graduate, you need to have some idea of what you want to do and some training to do it. Maybe just secretarial skills, typing and like that. Maybe an accounting course. Or computers. They are really important in any business these days."

"Yeah, but—"

Forks clattered onto plates as the tones went off. "Fairfax Police to Fairfax ambulance. The ambulance is needed for a person with difficulty breathing at 127 Forrest Court. The name is Van Mark."

Clyde swiveled his chair toward the radio and keyed

the mike. "10–4. 45–01 is responding to 127 Forrest Court, the Van Mark residence, for a person with difficulty breathing."

"Your time out is zero-eight-fourteen."

"So much for breakfast," Maryanne grumbled, stuffing one last bite of Clyde's superior mushroom and cheese omelet into her mouth and heading for the garage.

When they arrived at the Van Mark residence, they found that Peter Van Mark, a seventy-two-year-old emphysema patient, was indeed having trouble getting his breath. They placed him on oxygen and bundled him into the rig for the fifteen-minute trip down Route 10 to Fairfax General. As they started toward the hospital, Maryanne noticed that Peter's lips were becoming blue despite the oxygen constantly feeding his non-rebreather mask.

"Rose," she called through the small window between the box and the driver's seat, "let's take this code 3 to avoid the morning traffic."

Rose knew that Maryanne's upbeat comment had an underlying seriousness to it. Maryanne would never use the siren just to avoid traffic. Without alarming the patient, she was telling Rose that Mr. Van Mark's condition was becoming more serious. "Sure, no problem," she said, and almost immediately the wail of the siren began to fill the air.

"I had a girl in my class named Van Mark," Kate said to Peter. "Did someone in your family graduate from Fairfax High last year?"

The man beamed. "Why, yes," he said, his voice slightly muffled by the mask, "that would be my granddaughter Carla." His sentences came out in short bursts as he struggled to get his breath. Maryanne might have asked Kate not to talk to him to avoid tiring him, but his mental attitude was important too, and Kate certainly seemed to be cheering him up.

"Right," Kate said. "Carla. That was it. She wasn't in any of my classes but I knew of her." Always considerate of the patients, Kate took Peter's hand. "She was really pretty."

While the two talked, Maryanne, on the small jump seat at the patient's head, began the paperwork and Clyde prepared to move to Kate's side on the crew bench so he could get another set of vitals.

T.C. Stevens was late for work. Impatiently, leaving one hand on the steering wheel, he grabbed his cup of coffee from the holder beside his elbow and slugged down a large swallow. "Shit," he muttered, blowing thick streams of air between his teeth. "Hot." Rubbing his stinging tongue on the roof of his mouth, he slowed at the stop sign at the intersection of Route 10 and heard the siren. He looked to his right and saw the approaching ambulance. Although he was just a few feet from the stop sign, his Chevy had slowed only to about fifteen miles per hour. Usually he didn't have to stop but merely make the right he needed to head for the parkway. As he saw the white-and-orange vehicle speeding toward him, lights flashing and siren wailing, he worried about sliding into the intersection. He slammed his foot down on the brake pedal, causing the coffee to slosh over the rim of the cup and into his lap. Yelping, he tried to brush the burning liquid from his pants and upper thighs, his attention no longer focused on his driving. As he jerked, his foot moved from the brake to the gas. Realizing that his car was still drifting into the intersection, he slammed the pedal down.

Rose had been wearing her seat belt, but that didn't protect her from the impact that forced the driver's door against her left hip. Reflexively she slammed the brake as the ambulance was pushed sideways. Her head rattled first left, then right, then left again. Trying to comprehend what had just happened, she looked to her left and saw the small black vehicle now crushed against the side of the rig. She picked up the mike. "45–01. Been hit. Accident. Main and Route 10. Get an ambulance here." Then, with tears running down her face and a severe pain in her left side, she dropped the mike onto the seat beside her and concentrated on trying to keep from panicking.

In the back everything that wasn't inside a compartment suddenly became a projectile. A stethoscope, BP cuff, pens, and a flashlight flew around. Cabinets sprang and everything from soft trauma dressings to quart containers of sterile water careened around the inside of the rig. Maryanne had been holding the metal box that the crew used for the PCR, but on impact it was jerked from her hands and struck Kate in the forehead. Clyde, who had been changing position at the time of impact, was thrown against the far wall, then landed on top of the patient. The side of Maryanne's head slammed into the wall of the rig and she was knocked unconscious. As the vehicle rocked, more cabinet doors flew open, dumping linen, heavy containers of water-gel blankets, and oxygen masks over the victims.

When Rose hit the brake, the rig stopped suddenly and the car behind, a small Geo Metro that had been following too closely, slammed into its back end, springing the back doors and dumping a hodgepodge of first-aid supplies onto the roadway.

I had been starting a load of laundry when I heard the original call. I'd listened as the crew picked up the patient and called in that it was on its way to the hospital. After about five minutes of quiet, I heard Rose's jumbled call for help. I was on the phone immediately.

"Fairfax Police," Mark Thomas said.

"Did I hear right?" I asked. "It's Joan. Has the ambulance been in an accident?"

"We don't have confirmation, but we heard what you heard. She said Main and Route 10. We've got two cars on the way. Maybe you'd better head over there."

"I'm on the way. Just in case, tone out for a driver to pick up another rig and an attendant."

"Sure thing, Joan. Whoever gets there first can let us know."

I grabbed my portable radio and my police scanner so I would be able to hear the responding police vehicles and ran for my car. As I drove I heard Mark toning out for a driver and an attendant.

The location of the reported accident was only about a mile from my house. As I approached, I heard Eileen Flynn's very excited voice say, "The ambulance has been in an accident. We've got numerous injuries. Send two ambulances for starters. I'll update you."

"10–4, Eileen. Joan Lloyd's on the way and I've got crew for one rig. I'll tone out for a second."

Traffic was at a complete standstill, but with my green light flashing and an occasional honk, I was able to drive along the shoulder of Route 10 until I got to within a few car lengths of the accident. I stopped, grabbed a pair of gloves, and ran. Puffing, I could see that the rig and a car behind it were crumpled.

"God, Joan, am I glad to see you," Eileen said as I approached.

"What do you know so far?" I asked Eileen.

"Very little. One car broadsided the rig. The guy's hurt pretty bad." She pointed as she talked. "This car hit the rig from behind, but they're not too bad. I haven't been inside the ambulance yet."

"Do what you can, and I'll see what's inside the rig. And get the fire department here, if only for manpower."

Eileen looked a bit wide-eyed. She was a good cop and very helpful in EMS situations, but this was quite a bit over her head. Actually it was over my head too, but I fell back on the basic principles. You can't treat what you don't know about, I had taught in my classes. If you're alone, your first job is to find out *how many* and *how bad*. "Just do the best you can," I said. She nodded and walked around the side of the rig toward the front. "And have them put the helicopter on standby," I yelled at her back. I saw her key her portable radio and knew that my requests would be relayed to the police dispatcher.

I took a deep breath and walked up to the rear of the ambulance. Triage. There were more patients than care-givers, and since I was the only functioning EMT around, I needed to assess and prioritize the injuries so we could treat the most serious, but salvageable ones, first.

I looked inside and tried to separate the patients from the chaos. On quick inspection I saw Clyde, awkwardly draped over the patient, who had been sitting upright on the stretcher. Kate lay on the crew bench, blood pouring from a long and deep laceration on her head, and Maryanne was slumped over in the crew seat, still in her seat belt.

I started with the two people on the stretcher. Clyde was lying across the patient's lap. "Clyde," I said softly. "Are you all right?"

"I think my leg's broken. It got twisted when I fell. My back hurts like hell too."

"Fingers and toes wiggle?" I asked him.

"Yeah. That's the first thing I checked. But I can't move without a lot of pain. My breathing's okay and my pulse is strong. I'm really scared and I can't get off this poor man without help."

"Got it." Okay, I told myself, he's conscious and alert. For the moment category yellow, a serious injury but he could wait. "Sir," I said to the man seated on the stetcher, "how are you doing?"

"I can't find my mask," he said, his breathing shallow and rapid. "It got knocked off."

"I'll find it for you," I said.

"It's here," Clyde said, slowly reaching beneath him with as little movement as possible and handing the oxygen mask to the older man.

"Your name, sir?" I asked as I listened to the hiss of the flowing oxygen.

"Peter," the dazed man said.

"Okay, Peter, just hold on for a moment." I scooped some of the debris from the floor and climbed into the ambulance. I helped Peter grasp the mask and he pressed it against his face, gasping for oxygen. His lips were blue and he was sweating profusely. Triage red, I thought. He'll be one of the first transported. Trying to help him relax, I added, "You'll just have to put up with Clyde there in your lap for a few minutes. Is that okay? He's a nice enough fellow."

"Sure," Peter said, gently patting Clyde on the back.

I climbed around Clyde and touched Kate's shoulder. "Hi, Kate," I said. "How's the head?"

"It hurts a lot," she said, "and I think I broke my arm, but the rest of me's okay."

"Did you lose consciousness at any time?"

"No. I'm okay. But check Maryanne. She's totally out."

"Good girl. Hang in there." Triage yellow, or even green. She could wait until I had lots more manpower. Ankle deep in equipment and supplies, I finally maneuvered around to Maryanne and placed one hand on either side of her head. "Can you hear me?" I asked softly. I didn't want her jerking awake and moving her head or neck.

She moaned but didn't open her eyes. "Maryanne?"

I got no response. Okay, I thought to myself, she's in serious condition and she'll need quick treatment. At a minimum I've got two reds, Maryanne and Peter, and two yellows, Kate and Clyde. The guy that Eileen said was in bad shape is probably another red. At least three ambulances, if we can get them, and the helicopter. I opened the side door of the rig and climbed out. "Just a few minutes, everyone. I'll be right back."

Although I wanted to treat my patients, that couldn't be my first priority. Before I could concentrate on any one victim, I had to be sure that the right number of ambulances were responding and I had to assess the rest of the accident victims.

I keyed my mike. "45–24 to FPD."

"PD on. Go ahead, 45–24."

"Have them launch the chopper. In addition, so far I need a total of at least three rigs. Call Prescott and whoever else you need and get manpower here ASAP."

"10–4, Joan. Prescott's sending two rigs and I've got Jack McCaffrey picking up 45–02, and Jill Tremonte and Ed Herman responding to the scene. Nick Abrams is on the way to pick up –03. That gives you four ambulances responding."

"Tone out again and get any available manpower from FVAC to the scene. Is the fire department responding with manpower and their rescue?"

"10–4 to that, Joan."

I sighed. Although not an ambulance, the fire department's rescue truck contains oxygen cylinders, extra backboards, and other immobilization equipment we'd need until other ambulances arrived. "Great. I'll get you more information when I have it." I took a deep breath. My heart was pounding and adrenaline was pumping through my body. I had to calm down and use my brain, not my muscles. I took another deep breath to further clear my head and ease my shaking hands.

"Lady," someone yelled from beside the passenger door of the tiny bright green Metro now about three feet from the rig's back doors. "You gotta fix my wife. She's bleeding all over the place."

"I'll take a look." I walked over and looked at the woman seated in the passenger seat. She had a long gash on her right forearm and she was crying loudly. Good breathing, I thought. "Ma'am," I said loudly over her wails, "what hurts?"

"My arm. My arm. I'm bleeding."

"I see. Do you hurt anywhere else?"

"No, but there's blood."

"I know. Do you remember the accident?"

"Yeah. That damned ambulance stopped for no reason."

For the moment she was a triage category green. The

moderate bleeding was controlled and she had no other obvious injuries. Every patient would be reevaluated when I had the personnel, but for now she could wait.

"And, sir, how are you?"

"I'm okay, but you gotta help her," her husband screamed, grabbing my jacket.

"Right now I have others who need my help more than your wife. Just be patient."

"Patient? She's bleeding." He held onto my jacket.

"Sir. If you don't let me go I'll have you restrained by the police."

"But she's bleeding."

Already sweating from the combination of adrenaline and exertion, I slipped my arms out of my jacket and walked away, leaving the amazed man still holding onto the sleeve.

Shaking my head, I walked around the intertwined black-and-white vehicles. I saw that Eileen was with the driver of the Chevy so I continued to the driver's side window of the ambulance. The door was going to need to be opened with the jaws since the small car was pressed up against it. Someone had broken out all the glass. "Rose," I said. "How are you doing?"

"I think I'm okay but I'm stuck here. My feet are tangled in the pedals and this door is jammed."

"Are you hurt?"

"I'm not really sure. I've got some pain in my side but I'm certainly not in the first batch to be transported since they will have to cut me out of here. How's Maryanne?"

"She's unconscious, Kate's got a head laceration and a possible broken arm, and Clyde's draped across the patient's lap. He looks pretty ridiculous."

Rose smiled weakly. "It wasn't my fault."

"I know," I said.

"I had my lights and siren going."

"I know." I squeezed her shoulder gently. "Try to relax and I'll be back."

"Okay. But it wasn't my fault."

Eileen tapped me on the shoulder. "The driver over here's pretty bad. He's got memory loss and keeps fading out on me."

I walked over and focused on the driver of the Chevy. "Sir. How are you doing?"

"What happened?"

"You had an accident. Where do you hurt?"

"Hurt? Everywhere." He sounded bewildered. He looked at me. "Who are you?"

"I'm with the ambulance corps. What hurts worst?"

"Hurts? What happened? Who are you?" It was a cool fall day and he was shivering violently.

Okay, I thought to myself. Short-term memory loss, probably a head injury. He's a red and Rose is a green, or maybe a yellow. I looked at Eileen and motioned to the Chevy's driver. "Is he entangled?"

"I don't think so," she said. The fire department wouldn't have to cut him out of his car. "I checked his legs and he seems free. Rose will need to be cut out though. I need to flare all this out."

"I know. Good job. Go." I counted on my fingers. We had at least three reds, two yellows, and at least two greens, counting the passenger in the Metro. I wasn't sure about her husband yet. I walked around to the rear of the ambulance where I would set up a small control area and keyed my mike again. "45–24 to FPD."

"PD on."

"Updated count. Write this down. We have three reds,

two yellows, and two, possibly three greens. Get someone on the phone to Fairfax General, the trauma center, and, if needed, whatever other hospitals you can and see what room they have, and have them gear up for our arrival. We'll update them on exact numbers as we load patients. And see whether the chopper can take two." Depending on which helicopter was responding to our scene, it could take either one or two of my reds.

I glanced at my watch. Everything I had done so far had taken less than three minutes. Out of the corner of my eye I saw the fire department rescue truck arrive, and several cars with blue lights had pulled up behind my car.

Chief Bradley ran up to me. "What's the situation, Joan?"

"Well, Chief, the ambulance driver will have to be extricated, but you'll have to let me know whether we need to get the guy out of the Chevy first. Most of all I need hands."

"Sure, Joan. Use what you need." He turned. "Mike, Harry, get over here."

Two firemen with whom I had worked before ran up. "Guys," I said, "I need one person with the Chevy driver. He's got an altered mental status and needs to be kept still to avoid compromising any neck or head injury. Another can hold head stabilization on Maryanne. When I checked she was unconscious in the rig. And use gloves." I deployed another firefighter to check the occupants of every car that had even been tapped to see whether anyone else would need transport, and one more to assemble backboards, immobilization equipment, and blankets in a single location so we could get to equipment efficiently. "And oxygen cylinders and masks. See whether you can use the trauma bags or cylinders from this rig. Scavenge what you can."

I was incredibly relieved to hear the siren of an approaching ambulance. Eileen and Chuck Harding had stopped all traffic on both Route 10 and Main Street and had put flares everywhere. The approaching ambulance wove around lines of stopped cars and pulled up in the oncoming traffic lane. Jill and Jack climbed out.

"What can we do, Joan?" Jack asked.

God, was I glad to see them. Now, where to put two EMTs? Jack was the more experienced. "Jack, take the man in the black Chevy. We'll need to immobilize him whatever way you think is best. He's a red, with altered mental status. I haven't done any survey or vitals." He disappeared around the side of the rig.

Jill was relatively new and had a bit of a deer-in-the-headlights look. Specific tasks, I said to myself. "Jill, first pull all the trauma bags and MCI kits off of 45–02 and stack them in an equipment staging area wherever you think it will work. One of the firefighters has started but you'll know better exactly what we'll need. And blankets and splints," I added. "Then see whether you can have someone put each patient in the rig on oxygen and maybe in a collar if possible. The patient on the stretcher's name is Peter and he's having severe respiratory difficulty, or was when I was last in there. See that he's got enough oxygen."

"I'll do what I can, Joan."

As she turned I squeezed her upper arm and smiled. "I know you'll do fine."

More help was arriving every minute, firefighters, engines, police cars, but not what I wanted to see most—

more EMTs. I sighed. It was Wednesday morning and there were few people around.

I keyed my mike again. "45–24 to FPD."

"PD's on, Joan. Go ahead."

"What's the status of responding ambulances?"

"Prescott's got two crews and is en route with two rigs. Your second rig should be there already. And the chopper's got an ETA of five minutes and can only carry one. Your third rig hasn't called in that it's responding yet."

I counted again. The Chevy driver would go in the chopper. Maryanne and Peter would be transported by the first two rigs, ours and Prescott's first rig, with the woman with the cut arm in one if the EMT in charge agreed that they could handle both a red and a green. That left Kate, Clyde, and Rose and any more walking wounded who decided that they were hurt later. People often complained of delayed symptoms, either of real injuries or from cases of Allstate-itis.

We'd need at least one more ambulance or one would have to come back to the scene from the hospital and pick up more patients. I wanted Maryanne to go to the trauma center, but Peter would be just as well off at FGH so the rig that took him there could do a quick turn-around. Or maybe the chopper could do a hot off-load—remove one patient with the blades still turning, hand off to the ER staff, and return for another. I'd have to talk to them about it.

As I prepared to climb back into the ambulance to reassess the patients, I spotted Ed's little Neon. Never was I more glad to see him.

"Ed," I shouted as I watched him get out of his car.

"See about Rose, in the driver's seat. If she's okay, come into the back and help me."

He nodded and moved away.

"Lady," the husband of the woman with the arm laceration yelled, "you gotta help my wife. She's in pain." He strode up to me, fire in his eye.

"Sir," I said, mustering all the patience I had, "there are several critical injuries here. Your wife can wait and *will* wait."

"But—"

"Sir. Would you like me to let someone die so I can fix your wife's boo-boo?" He was silent as I turned and climbed into the back of the ambulance. I was able to get more into patient care, now that I had capable hands tending to the other wounded. I would begin with Clyde.

I had been at the post office, almost ten minutes away, when I had heard Rose's original call for help. I had phoned the police quickly and started toward the scene in my Neon. As I drove toward Route 10, trying not to push the car any faster than I could drive safely, I heard Joan's initial reports. Still about four minutes from the scene, I heard her increasing level of tension, telling me that she was coping but without enough capable help.

I pulled up behind a line of blue-lighted firefighters' cars and saw Joan behind the ambulance. I could see that the back of it had been hit, and I also noted the small black Chevy embedded in the driver's side.

"Ed," she yelled at me, "see about Rose, in the driver's seat. If she's okay, come into the back and help me."

I walked around the passenger side of the ambulance and carefully opened the undamaged passenger side door. "Hi, Rose," I said. "I hear you've had an accident."

She smiled weakly. "Ed. I'm so glad you're here. Joan was here a few minutes ago and I told her I was okay." She hesitated. "But I can't feel my feet."

Oh shit, I said to myself. "Okay, Rose. Let me check you over." I scrunched down, around the crushed metal that held Rose in her seat, and found her right foot. I squeezed her toes. "Can you feel that?"

"Somewhat, but it's fuzzy like."

"Okay. Can you move those toes?"

She moved them, but only a little. "It hurts in my back really bad when I even try," she said, tears now rolling freely down her face. "And my chest hurts when I take a deep breath. My whole left side actually."

There was a wide console between the two front seats, filled with controls for the lights and siren, the two-way radio, and a scanner. I climbed onto it and placed my hand in the center of Rose's chest. "Take a deep breath, Rose," I said.

She inhaled. I could feel her chest rise evenly. I grabbed the stethoscope that was looped around my neck and placed the diaphragm on the right side of her chest, just below her collarbone. "Another deep breath, Rose," I said. As I listened I could hear normal sounds at the apex of her right lung. I repeated the process on the left side. Everything appeared to be normal. Satisfied that there was no immediate threat to her breathing, I said, "I'm going to find the fire department so we can get you out of here. I'll be right back."

"Promise?" she asked, her voice tiny and obviously frightened.

"Promise."

I ran around to the back of the ambulance and peered

inside. "Joan," I said, "Rose is a red. Have you got enough rigs for that?"

"Red?" Joan looked puzzled.

"Is she that bad?" Clyde asked.

I didn't want to give detailed answers. "She's got some neurological deficit and a chest injury. She's stable now but I think she needs to be treated as soon as the fire department can get her out."

"Okay," Joan said. "We're still short of transportation. I'll call the police and see whether there are any more rigs within ten minutes. I gather that Davenport's having trouble raising a crew since they're out on one call already. We've got a total of four ambulances and the chopper responding."

"It will take the fire department a while to get Rose out so she can go in a late-arriving ambulance," I said, "or even on a turnaround."

"Right."

"If you don't need me here, I'll get back to Rose."

Joan and I looked into the back of the ambulance. Jill was bandaging Kate's head laceration. A firefighter was holding Maryanne's head. It was ordered, crowded chaos. "We're okay back here for now and Jack's with the Chevy guy."

Pam Kovacs's Bronco pulled to a stop at the back of the line of cars parked on the shoulder. As she ran up, Joan said, "You take care of Rose, Ed. Pam can help Jack with the driver."

"Great. I promised her I'd be right back." I grabbed an oxygen tank and a non-rebreather mask from the pile of equipment at the rear of the rig and walked back to the passenger side of the ambulance. As I slid in beside Rose, I saw Nick Abrams park 45–03 beside –02.

"Looks like we've got an army," Rose said.

"Yeah, and now I can stay with you." I connected the oxygen and slipped the mask over Rose's face. Then I pressed her forehead gently against the headrest to stabilize her head. "Just don't move."

"Hey," she said, "I'm a better EMT than that. I haven't moved a bit." She remembered looking over at the Chevy. "Well, almost."

I smiled. "Good girl."

As we sat, I watched Jack and Pam begin to package the Chevy driver. "He just slammed into me," Rose said softly. "I couldn't help it."

"I know that, Rose. You're a fine driver."

"I just caught a glimpse of the car out of the corner of my eye, but by then I couldn't get out of the way." A tear rolled down her cheek. "It seemed like he sped up and hit me full force."

She started to turn her head to watch what was going on in the Chevy, but I held her still. "No moving, remember?"

She smiled weakly. "Right. What's going on? Is he real bad?"

"I can't really tell," I said. "They've got him in a collar and they're doing a rapid extrication. From the look of the windshield, he hit his head. No seat belt."

Rose reached up and patted the shoulder harness. "Don't leave home without it. How about the guys in the back?"

"I don't know very much," I said.

Rose gently reached over and turned up the rig's scanner. "I want to listen now. Before it was just too loud and too confusing." As the babble filled the front seat, we just became quiet and listened. "And maybe we can hear them call the hospital. That way we'll know about everyone else," Rose added.

"21–01 is 10–19," someone on the scanner said.

"That's one of Prescott's rigs," I said. "It sounds like Les Kravitski."

"I forget you ride with Prescott too."

"Yeah, and Joan too now."

"Air One to ground. We're one minute out. LZ still unchanged?"

"10–4, Air One."

"I wonder where they're landing the chopper," Rose said.

"Right on Route 10, if they can, I assume. That way we won't have to tie up a vehicle to transport someone to the chopper."

At that moment, Chief Bradley arrived at Rose's window. "Hi, Rose," he said. "The jaws are here and we'll have you out in a jiffy."

"Great, Chief," Rose said. "But exactly how long is a jiffy?"

It was just like Rose to try to be cheerful in a scary situation like this one. The chief grinned. "Slightly longer than a moment and shorter than a while."

Every time I tried to get into the rig to start to treat a patient, more decisions had to be made, so I situated myself beside the back doors. Now I had at least two rigs to transport patients and the helicopter would soon be ready to load. I wanted to try to keep 45–02 at the scene so we could scrounge additional equipment as it became necessary. Eileen Flynn walked up to the back of the ambulance where I was trying to keep everything straight in my head. "Joan," she said to me, "the chopper's almost down. They want to know who's going on it. Just so you know, the guy from the Chevy's unconscious now."

"He's going in the chopper. And Clyde and Peter here will be in the first two rigs, our −03 and the first Prescott rig. I would like to get Maryanne out next but it's such close quarters here that we've got to get those two out first in order to get to her."

"Okay. Prescott's second rig is about five minutes out and Davenport's about ten behind that."

Behind me, Jill and Nick had Clyde immobilized on a backboard and were finishing strapping him down. As they lowered him into the hands of several waiting firefighters, I said, "How's the back and the leg, buddy?"

"They hurt like hell. How's Rose? I heard Ed say she had some neuro problem."

"You know as much as I do right now, Clyde. Let's just get you going."

I had two rigs to choose from, but the decision was an easy one, the first easy one all day. "Put him in Prescott's rig. Then we can move the stretcher from this rig to our −03 with Peter still on it. Have them pull −03's stretcher out and just leave it here for now." As I watched, they loaded Clyde into Prescott's rig and, with the Prescott crew in charge, lights flashing and siren wailing, the ambulance drove off toward Fairfax General. Peter sat on the stretcher, clutching an oxygen mask against his face. He was now ashen and his fingertips were slightly bluish. He denied any neck or back injury, and, with his respiratory distress making it difficult for him to lie down, we decided that he would be better off without spinal immobilization.

We quickly unlocked the stretcher and lifted it down. We then rolled him to −03 and lifted him inside. With Jill in charge and Nick driving, the rig sped off toward Fairfax General Hospital.

As the two ambulances drove away, I saw several people carrying the Chevy driver to the helicopter, now on the ground about two hundred yards down Route 10. Okay, I told myself, three gone. Pam and Jack would quickly turn their patient over to the flight nurses and then would be able to help with Maryanne and Kate. I climbed back into the ambulance. Kate was now on the crew bench on a longboard with a collar around her neck and an oxygen mask over her face.

"I never realized how really uncomfortable this is," she said. "My back is killing me. And, just to remind you, I'll eventually need a splint for my arm."

I pushed the mess from the floor to where Peter's stretcher had been, and as it shifted I saw the familiar flash of bright orange. I reached down and came up brandishing a short splint. "It just so happens. . . ."

I found a roll of gauze and quickly affixed Kate's arm to the board. Then I unbuttoned the bottom buttons of her uniform shirt and pulled one tail from her pants. I folded it up over the arm and splint. Next I found a triangular bandage among the rubble and removed the packaging. Several safety pins fell out and I used them to pin the shirt tail down so her arm was tightly affixed to her chest. Then I used the hollow of her spine to slide one end of the folded triangular bandage beneath her and used it to bind her forearm tightly to her ribs.

"Thanks, that's really much better."

"I'm sorry about the backboard," I said.

"I know. It's okay."

Brenda Frost, who had arrived on Prescott's second rig, poked her head into the rig. "Hi, Joan. Fancy meeting you here. Just to let you know, our second rig's ready to transport," she said. "Who've we got?"

"Why don't you take Kate, here? She just needs some head blocks, straps, and tape and she's ready to go." We had all the equipment we needed now, so I could use our second rig for transport. "Then I can get Maryanne into –02." Unless the chopper could do a hot off-load.

"Sure thing," Brenda said. Quickly she and Les Kravitski got Kate ready to go.

Pam and Jack arrived and I directed them to Maryanne, still being held by a firefighter. "Can the chopper come back?" I asked Pam.

"They're not sure. They've got a priority neonatal transport already scheduled so they'll radio ground control and find out whether they can delay it."

I kept planning out loud to help me think. "If they can, then we can take Rose in –02, if it's got enough equipment left. Otherwise we can use the Davenport rig that's on the way or maybe –03 can do a quick turnaround."

"Hey, Joan," Brenda called as they lifted Kate from the damaged ambulance, "we can take a green if you've got any."

I suddenly remembered the woman with the arm injury.

"Let me see," I said, walking to the Geo. "Sir," I said to the woman's husband, now sitting in the driver's seat, "we can take your wife now." I saw that someone had bandaged her arm.

"That's all right. I'm sorry about before. She's really fine. She can wait. Just take care of the worse-off people."

"Did anyone talk to her about her condition?"

"Someone asked her a lot of questions while he bandaged her arm. He said she doesn't need to go to the hospital right away. But she will need stitches. She's really fine."

I talked to the woman for a moment and ascertained that she was, indeed, uninjured, except for her laceration. "I don't want any of that collar stuff," she said. "I'm really fine. I'll sign something if you need me to. That nice man said you might. I just want someone to look at my arm."

"If you're sure you have no pain in your neck or back, we won't immobilize you," I said. "You and your husband can go in that ambulance over there." I pointed to the rig into which they were loading Kate.

The man handed me my jacket. "I'm really sorry for getting so upset before."

"No problem. I understand. Stress does odd things to us all," I replied.

"Thank you," he said, then followed his wife to the waiting ambulance.

In the deafening roar of the helicopter's liftoff, I watched as the ambulance with Kate and the couple inside pulled away toward Fairfax Hospital.

Pam and Jack had already gotten Maryanne, still unconscious, onto a backboard and were finally carrying her from the wrecked ambulance to –02. Pam called to me over her shoulder. "We're going to the trauma center so we'll be gone awhile."

"Sure thing," I shouted. I had already called for a second Davenport ambulance to stand by in our headquarters; several other neighboring ambulance corps and rescue squads were also on standby in case Prescott or Fairfax had another call while we were all tied up at the accident.

Finally the only one left was Rose. I became aware of the noise of the jaws of life.

"Ed," Rose said to me, "I really can't feel my feet."

"It will be just another minute or two," I said, warm and sweating beneath the tarp that Chief Bradley had draped over us. "They've got the door off and now they're pulling back a section of the side panel. You're just about out of here."

My shoulders ached from having held my hand against Rose's forehead for all this time, but I knew I could hang on a bit longer. "How are your grandchildren?"

"Davy's almost four and a holy terror," she yelled. Between her oxygen mask and the din of the jaws we could barely communicate, but we both kept talking anyway. I leaned my ear close to her mouth. "And Peggy's two and somehow manages to strain everything she eats through everything she wears."

"We've got it," someone yelled. "She's free."

I felt the tarp lifted from our heads and breathed in the suddenly cool air. Joan arrived at the driver's opening. "We've got a board all ready, and by the time you're ready to go –03 will be back from the hospital."

With extreme care, we removed Rose from the twisted metal and immobilized her on a longboard. "Okay, Rose," I said, placing my fingers in her hands, "let's check you out. Hold my hands and squeeze." She did. Hard. "Good girl. Sensations okay there?"

"Yes," she said.

"Take a deep breath. Any pain?"

"My left ribs. And I can feel something grating."

"Okay," I said. "Let's check your feet." I squeezed the big toe on her right foot. "Feel this?"

"Yeah. Actually I do." She grinned.

"That's fantastic." I squeezed her left. "And that?"

"Yeah. Maybe I'm okay after all."

"It sure seems so."

A few hours later, Joan and I sat around the table at headquarters with several of the people who had been on the call. We looked at the PCRs all arrayed on the table. Amazed, Joan said, "From the time of the call to Rose's arrival at the hospital was only thirty-three minutes. I'm flabbergasted. In some ways it felt like hours and in some it felt like only moments."

"I don't know whether I could have handled it," Nick said.

"You would have done whatever you could, just like I did," she said.

I took her hand. "You were great."

The phone rang and Jill picked it up, listened, then hung up. "Okay, here's the latest from Fairfax General. Rose had a fractured L4 and some serious sprains in her neck, but the doctor said that she'll have no neurological deficit. She's also got three broken ribs."

L4, the fourth lumbar vertebra. Broken. She's lucky that her spinal cord wasn't injured.

"And Kate is doing fine," Jill continued. "Just a broken arm and eight stitches in her head. I gather that was from the PCR box. She'll be kept overnight just to be sure. Peter, the original patient, is in the cardiac care unit. He was having a heart attack."

"How's Clyde?" Joan asked.

"Clyde's right tibia is broken but the rest of him's fine. It was a clean break so they think they can avoid surgery. And the lady's arm took twenty-seven stitches."

Nick whistled. "I bandaged it. She was making light of it. That must have been one long, deep sucker. But she kept apologizing and checking to be sure that I wasn't needed for someone more serious."

"That was me," Joan said, and repeated her encounter with the woman's husband. "Finally he seemed to understand, but I'm sorry I corked off at him."

"Sounds like he asked for it," I said.

"Phew," Pam said, walking into the kitchen. "What a morning."

"How's Maryanne?"

"She regained consciousness in the rig on the way to the trauma center. She's got a concussion and they're keeping her for a day or so. She's got no memory of anything this morning at all. But her vision and all her neurological functions are okay."

"That's great news. Did you happen to find out about the driver of the car that hit the rig?"

"Open head injury. And, for some reason, first- and mild second-degree burns on his thighs and in his groin. He's expected to pull through."

"Well, guys," I said, standing up. "Now the hard part. We've got –02 restocked and pretty much cleaned up, but we need to work on –03."

Jill stood up. "I think I hear my mother calling me."

"Not a chance," Joan said, getting to her feet. "We were all in this together earlier, we're all in this together now. Let's do it. But one last thing. If anyone needs to talk to someone about this, like the CISD team, please let the captain know and he'll set up a debriefing."

"Yeah," Jill said, "it might be good. It was really tough working on friends. I've never worked on someone I knew before."

"Me neither," Pam said, "but I've been to a Critical Incident Stress Debriefing before. It really helped just to talk about things. Actually I'll never forget it."

Pam's ambulance call had happened on a Tuesday afternoon. The following Thursday evening a group of people who had responded to the call gathered at FVAC headquarters. Seated around a long table in the meeting room were eight people. On one side of the table sat Ivan Zimberoff and three members of the stress debriefing team. Facing them sat four of the twelve people who had been involved in the rescue. None of the firefighters and only one of the police officers had accepted the invitation to the debriefing session.

"Why don't we start by introducing ourselves," Ivan began. "I'll start and then we'll go around the table counterclockwise. My name's Ivan and in addition to being the head of this team, I'm both an EMT and a volunteer firefighter."

Ivan was followed by each member of the debriefing team: an EMT, another firefighter, and a police officer. All of them had been trained in stress-resolving techniques and were there as much for support as for having had any special psychological training. Years earlier it had been discovered that many good professionals in EMS, police, and firefighting were being lost every year to what was called posttraumatic stress. States and counties began to adopt plans to try to deal with stress quickly after a serious accident, before the sleep disorders, personality changes, and other symptoms could progress and become serious psychological problems. They had learned that what was most needed was to give those involved in a difficult call the ability to share and verbalize their feelings.

After each member of the team had introduced himself, each of the people who had been at the accident scene gave their name and affiliation.

"Okay. What I'd like to do now," Ivan said, "is go around again. This time I'd like each person who responded to the accident to tell what he or she was doing when the call came in and what he or she did at the accident scene."

Phil Ortiz spoke first, fiddling with a keychain-flashlight. "Well, I was hanging out here at FVAC headquarters watching TV when the call came in for a PIAA on Julie Street near the intersection with Overlook Terrace. The dispatcher told me to respond to the scene but not to attempt to enter the vehicle until the fire department stabilized it. Then Pam called in and said that she would respond directly to the scene." He turned the tiny flashlight on and off as he spoke. "I radioed the police and told them that I would respond with the rig and that they should tone out for a third crew member.

"When I got to the scene, I was pretty shocked to see the front end of the car hanging over the embankment. The fire engine had just arrived and I could see firefighters pulling a line out from the winch to hook under the car and pull it away from the edge of the drop-off. I saw Pam and Chuck Harding standing at the back of the car, looking in, so I went over to them. Then I heard the guy inside the car yelling. I asked Chuck what was going on and he told me that we couldn't do anything until the car was secured." On and off the light flashed in Phil's hand.

"While the three of us stood and watched the car being

pulled away from the edge of the embankment, Heather showed up. When the firefighters had stabilized the car, we were able to gain entry. The car was a hatchback and the guy was crumpled in the well behind the seats. I crawled into the back and popped the hatch open. We were able to get him out pretty quickly after that. I drove to the hospital. We were about halfway to the trauma center when Pam yelled at me to radio the trauma center and let them know that we were coming in with a code. Then she shouted, 'Move your ass and get us there stat.' I looked in the rearview mirror, which, in an ambulance lets you see from the driver's seat into the back, and saw that Pam and Heather were doing CPR. I couldn't really go any faster if they were going to do effective CPR so I just continued." Realizing that he had been blinking his flashlight, he looked around the table and put the light down.

"Guess that's about it. We hung around the ER while they worked the guy, but the ER doc called it about twenty minutes after we got there."

Heather Franks was next. "I was all the way on the other side of town, at the Prescott A&P, when the pager tones on my portable radio went off. I pulled the portable out of my back pocket and called in. I told the dispatcher that I would respond but my ETA would be about fifteen minutes. Then I abandoned my grocery cart, hoping that it would still be there when I got back from the call, ran out to my car, and headed for Fairfax."

She sipped her coffee and continued. "By the time I got to the scene, the car had been stabilized and we were able to begin our extrication. The extrication was difficult because the guy was screaming and combative, but we got him out in about ten minutes. Once we completely immobilized him and got him into the rig, I checked his vitals while Pam did a complete survey. His vitals were within normal limits and he was responsive. He had also calmed down a lot. But about two or three minutes after we started toward the trauma center, he started to go out on us. His respirations became shallow and went up to about 40."

She again sipped her coffee. "Pam yelled at me to start bagging him while she took another BP. I grabbed the BVM and started to assist his breathing. Pam seemed frantic. She kept inflating the BP cuff and listening with her stethoscope. Then she tore the BP cuff off the guy's arm and threw it at me. She yelled, 'This fuckin' thing's not working,' and screamed at me to get her another one. I was a little worried about her. Pam's always so calm and in control, even in the most difficult situations." She looked at Pam, sitting beside her, quietly doing the needlepoint that always seemed to be in her hands.

"We were about halfway to the trauma center when I realized that the guy was no longer breathing on his own. I stopped bagging him for a few seconds to be sure, and Pam seemed to become even more frantic. 'Why the hell did you stop bagging him?' she yelled at me. I told her that I wanted to check whether he was breathing on his own. I placed my hand on his neck to check his carotid pulse and moved my hand around for a few seconds but I couldn't feel any pulse.

"I sort of took over after that. I told Pam to start CPR while I hooked our patient up to the cardiac monitor. It only took about a minute to turn on the machine and attach the electrodes to the guy's chest. I told Pam to stop CPR and then we both stared at the monitor screen. The monitor showed a flat line. Not even v-fib, just flatline.

'Oh my God,' Pam said, 'he's dead.' Then she yelled to Phil to step on it and get us to the hospital fast.

"Pam and I have worked a lot of codes together and I had never seen her react like that. I calmly told her to start compressions and said that I would ventilate. We did what we could but the ride seemed to take forever." Again Heather looked at Pam, but Pam's gaze was fixed on her needlepoint.

"After we got to the hospital," Heather continued, "Pam wouldn't move from the ER room where the trauma team was working our patient until the physician called the code. Phil and I made up the stretcher and replaced the BVM and the large shocking electrodes that we had used. As we wheeled the stretcher out of the ER, we saw Pam sitting on the curb next to the rig, just staring into space. She wouldn't talk to us, then or during the trip back to Fairfax. When we dropped her off at her car, she just jumped into the car, without a word to us, and drove away."

Pam was sitting next to Heather at the table, but when her turn to talk came, she just continued to stare at her needlepoint, the needle going through the coarse fabric with a smooth rhythm. "Pam," Ivan said. "Would you like to share your experience with us?"

Pam looked up. "Not right now," she answered. She turned toward Chuck, who was sitting on her right. "You go ahead, Chuck. I'll go after you."

Chuck Harding was wearing a sweatshirt with the words Fairfax Police Department on the front. "I had just started my shift when I was dispatched to a reported PIAA with possible entrapment," he began. "It took me about two minutes to get to the scene. When I got there I saw Pam's car with its green light flashing and the wrecked car with its front end hanging over the embankment. I pulled up behind Pam's Bronco and, as I got out of my patrol car, I could see her trying to get the rear hatch open. It scared the shit out of me because I could see that the car was rocking with her every move. It looked like it was about to go over the drop-off and take Pam with it. I ran over to her, grabbed her arm, and pulled her away from the vehicle. She yelled at me that there was an elderly man trapped inside and that he was badly injured.

"I was afraid that any attempt to get the hatch open would send the vehicle over the embankment so I wouldn't let her continue. I almost had to physically restrain her. I radioed headquarters to make sure that the fire department had been dispatched, then there was nothing that Pam or I could do but stand there and listen to the man scream. He was pleading for help, but there was really nothing that we could do. I know it was only a short time until the fire engine got to the scene and only another few minutes until they had the vehicle stabilized, but it seemed like forever. The man was screaming constantly all that time."

"When the call came in I was driving down Oak Street," Pam began as soon as Chuck finished. With her needlepoint now lying in her lap, she continued. "I was less than a minute from the accident scene. I knew that I would be the first trained person there and that's always scary, but I was totally unprepared for what I found. I saw the car teetering on the edge of a thirty-foot drop-off and heard the man screaming as soon as I got out of my car. I grabbed my crash kit and oxygen tank. As I approached the driver's side of the car, I could see that the front end of it was demolished and the windshield was shattered with the star-shaped pattern usually made by the impact of a head."

She took a great breath. "When I looked into the car I saw that the steering wheel was bent, but at first I couldn't see the person who was screaming. Then I saw him crumpled in the hatch area behind the rear seats. He was lying in a pool of blood and was still bleeding badly from the nose and mouth. It appeared that he had been thrown forward and had broken the windshield with his head and had then bounced all the way into the back of the vehicle.

"He was begging for help. I yelled to him that I was coming to help him and then went around to the back of the car. I tried to open the hatch, but it was locked. I didn't realize that the car was rocking until I felt Chuck grab my arm and pull me away. He kept holding my arm as we stood there and waited for the fire engine to arrive. I know now that it was dumb, to try to get into the car before the fire department got there, but the man kept screaming and screaming, and we just stood there." She shuddered. "There was nothing we could do. Nothing." She paused and swallowed hard.

"I remember supervising the extrication and thinking that we had lost much too much time. Still, I couldn't believe it when he started to go sour on us in the rig. He couldn't crap out on us now." She turned from Chuck to Heather. "I guess I just lost it. I don't remember much of what happened after that. All I remember was that I wanted to go home and go to sleep and forget the whole nightmare." Heather reached over and patted Pam's hand softly, then Pam picked up her canvas and worked her needle in and out.

"Okay," Ivan said. "Now that you've all shared your

experiences with us, I'd like to go around the table again and this time, I'll ask you to describe what you *felt* during the call. You've described what you did and what happened around you, now I'd like you to tell us what happened inside of you. Would you like to start, Phil?"

"Sure," Phil replied. "I guess the main thing I felt when I pulled the rig up to the scene was surprise and amazement. I thought, How the hell did the guy get his car in that position and how the hell did he end up in the back of the car? It was frustrating to wait for the engine to pull the car back, but that took only a few minutes, and then I was busy helping with the extrication." He pulled the flashlight from his pocket and played with the chain. "You know how it is on a bad call. There's so much to do that you don't have time to feel much. The screaming and all the blood bothered me, but I've been on bad calls before, and I can handle them. The only thing that really kind of shook me up was when Pam yelled at me to 'step on it.' Pam is FVAC's first lieutenant, and she was my advisor when I was in the youth group here. She was even one of the instructors of my EMT course. It was hard to ignore her order, but she was the one who taught me that the safety of the crew is the driver's responsibility. I guess she taught me real well because I did disobey her order to 'step on it.' I felt real bad on the way back to headquarters, though. I thought she was pissed off at me for not speeding up when she told me to."

"Heather," Ivan said.

"I heard the fire department dispatched on my car scanner," Heather said, "so I knew the accident was serious. The drive to the scene seemed to take forever, and I was angry and frustrated by a guy in front of me who was driving at twenty miles an hour and wouldn't let me pass even though he obviously saw my green light. I saw him looking up at the rearview mirror. I wanted to say to him 'How would you like it if your child was injured and someone deliberately obstructed someone who was coming to help him?'

"But, once I got to the scene, this call didn't feel much different from any other vehicle extrication. I guess I was a little angry with the patient for screaming and fighting us. It made the extrication a lot more difficult. I was able to begin working on him as soon as I got to the scene, and for most of the time I was just too busy to feel much of anything."

She sipped at her now-cold coffee. "I felt bad that we lost the guy, but I thought that the call went well, all things considered. We did everything possible for him. After the call was over, I was more concerned about Pam than about anything else. I've never seen her react like she did."

Staring at her needlework, Pam nodded for Chuck to go ahead of her again. "When I pulled up to the scene and saw Pam's car already there," he began, "I felt a sense of relief. I guess I ought to be used to it by now, being a cop and all, but I still hate being the first one on the scene of a personal injury motor vehicle accident. There's not much I can do except give an injured person oxygen or start CPR if I have to. I knew that Pam is one of the best EMTs in Fairfax, and I felt that she could handle the medical situation while I flared out the road and controlled traffic. But when I saw her trying to open the hatch and that the car was rocking, I was afraid that the car would go over and take her with it. I wanted to help the guy, but there was nothing we could do. I felt so helpless.

"The rest of the day was pretty much of a washout for me. I'm used to acting, not standing around. I just couldn't get over that awful feeling of helplessness."

It was Pam's turn. Her needle still moving rhythmically, she began. "About a year ago a very close friend of mine was killed in a car crash. I learned from one of the paramedics at the scene that it took more than forty minutes to extricate her from the wreckage and that she was conscious and in terrible pain. She died en route to the hospital."

She put down her needle. "I kept seeing her as I was trying to get to the man in the car. I know it was only a few minutes, but it seemed like hours that Chuck and I waited until the fire truck came and stabilized the car. I've never felt so frustrated and helpless in my life. I felt like I was letting him down, like I wasn't doing my job. His screams were tearing me apart.

"After the call was over, I felt so ashamed that I had lost control like I did. I had yelled at Phil and at Heather and had screwed up the call big time. I'm an EMT instructor. I'm supposed to set an example."

As Pam began to cry, Heather reached over and took her hand. "You do set an example," Heather said, "by doing your best and by being a caring person."

"I was one of the chiefs at a house fire a few years ago," Bud Collier, a burly Oakmont firefighter who was one of the members of the debriefing team, said. "One of my firefighters brought out a badly burned child. My own one-year-old daughter had almost died a week earlier from dehydration caused by an intestinal infection. I fell apart and began crying like a baby. Then, after the fire was over I thought, What will my firefighters think of me? They'll think I'm a real wimp. I was surprised when a number of them told me that the same kind of thing had happened to them at one time or another."

"In the kind of emergency work that all of us who are here do," Ivan said, "we have to allow ourselves to be human—to have feelings and to make mistakes sometimes. I know it's a cliché, but sometimes we have to be reminded that none of us are perfect. People who are involved in emergency responses are used to acting. One of the hardest things for us to deal with is being helpless in a situation where we feel that we should be doing something. But sometimes there's nothing we can do.

"I'd like to go around one more time, and this time I'd like each of you to tell where you are now. How about you, Phil?"

"I'm okay now," Phil said, stuffing his keys back in his pocket. "I don't let these things bother me. I've been on lots of bad calls and sometimes I feel awful, but I just make myself forget about them. I think that there's no point in dwelling on stuff I can't change. But I'm real glad that Pam wasn't angry at me for ignoring her when she told me to step on it."

"And you, Heather?" Ivan asked.

"I guess I was lucky I arrived late and didn't have to stand around and wait like Chuck and Pam did. I'm all right now. I'm still a little concerned about Pam, though."

"How about you, Chuck?" Ivan asked.

"I've been pretty shook up by this call," Chuck replied. "I've been up a lot at night, thinking about it. I've talked about it with my wife, but it's hard sharing this kind of thing with someone who has never had this kind of experience. And cops don't talk about feelings very much. I think this session has helped a lot."

"And you, Pam?"

Pam smiled. "This session has been a great help to me. I almost didn't come because I was sure that everyone was disappointed in me. I was even thinking of quitting FVAC."

"Because you weren't perfect?" Ivan asked.

"Yeah. I guess. I feel a lot better about that part, but I think it's going to take me some time to get over the call itself. It helps to know that other people have reacted that way, though."

"Well, we all handle stressful situations in different ways," Ivan said. "Whatever works for you is okay. And time helps a lot."

Phil, Heather, Chuck, Pam, and the members of the debriefing team stood around and talked for a while after the session. Then, one by one, they left, ready to take their next emergency call.

Pam stood up in the kitchen and looked around at all the people who had been involved in the rescue from the ambulance accident. "Yeah, I think it will be a good idea to set up a CISD session. I'll call Ivan and set it up."

"But first," Joan said, "it's cleanup time."

Chapter 6

When I first moved to Fairfax in 1966 with my then-husband and two small children, I had little contact with the police. I remember one time when my back door was inadvertently left open the night we returned from vacation and a concerned neighbor, not knowing we were back, asked the police to investigate. A pleasant officer showed up at my open door yelling "Hello?" When I arrived at the door, he merely assured himself that we were, indeed, the owners of the dwelling while my children, then preschoolers, looked on wide-eyed.

A few years later I was involved in my only auto accident in Fairfax and, since neither the driver of the other vehicle nor I was injured, a grumbling officer said only "Just move the car out of the intersection, lady." Of course I did.

Ed had different dealings with the police through his longtime service with FVAC. He developed a rapport with some and just tried to ignore the rest, a few old-timers whose sole interaction with the FVAC volunteers was to grumble "Just get these people out of the intersection." It took quite a while before FVAC managed to convince the police officers that EMTs do more than "you call, we haul."

Now the Fairfax officers are almost all relatively young and happy to have jobs with a suburban police department. Unlike their big-city counterparts, the police in Fairfax don't usually deal with violent crime. They spend most of their time making traffic stops, investigating the frequent burglar alarms, unlocking cars for motorists who have left their keys inside, and checking on the welfare of the elderly parents of frightened grown children who haven't been able to contact a loved one for several days. They also respond to almost every ambulance call and fire investigation.

Occasionally, however, members of the FPD have to react to more stressful situations.

Melissa Flowers and John Kirkwood had met in middle school, dated through high school, and married three days after graduation. Theirs had been a stormy marriage at best. They fought, separated, reconciled, and separated again. The worst fights occurred because Melissa enjoyed flirting and John was terribly jealous. Whether Melissa flirted because she enjoyed it or because it annoyed John was never totally clear, but their friends had grown accustomed to watching the two of them storm out of a party or club, usually with John dragging Melissa by the wrist.

One evening they had spent some time at the Red Foxx Lounge, a local Fairfax bar, and Melissa had caught the eye of a nice-looking biker type. At twenty-four, she was shapely and enjoyed wearing tight, revealing miniskirts and low-cut blouses. That particular evening John simmered, then, about midnight, boiled over. "Keep your eyes to yourself, you bitch," he shouted at his wife.

"It's none of your goddamn business where I look," Melissa countered.

"It's my goddamn business because you're my wife and my wife can't look at other men."

Melissa looked at the biker and shrugged, then turned to John. "You're really a bastard, you know that?"

"Yeah,"—John grinned—"but I'm your bastard and you'll do as I say."

"Shit," Melissa hissed, and took a large swallow of her Bud Light.

"Let's get out of here," John said.

"I'm not ready yet." Melissa's eyes had drifted back to the biker, clearly admiring his massive forearms.

"You are ready now," John said, his voice low and menacing.

"Aw, come on, baby," Melissa said, stroking John's arm. "Just one more drink. I'll make it worth your while when we get home." She grabbed his thigh under the small table and squeezed.

Undeterred, John snapped, "Now!"

Melissa knew when she had pushed her husband far enough, so reluctantly she finished her beer and followed him out to the car.

All during the drive home, John berated his wife for "messin'" with the biker. And just as loudly, Melissa told him that she wasn't his property and she could look where she pleased. When they arrived at their rented apartment, the argument suddenly escalated from a simple shouting match. John slapped Melissa across her face. "That's for your lying mouth," he said.

"Bastard," Melissa hissed, wiping a small drop of blood from her cut lip. "You're such a shit."

"And you're a slut," John said. "I don't know why I keep you around."

"*You* keep *me* around? Who earns more money? Tell me that."

John drew his arm back and, as Melissa ducked, his fist grazed the top of her head. Melissa was shocked. It was the first time that John had used his fist rather than just an open hand. Without thinking, she slammed a punch into his stomach.

The fight was on. After a few punches, Melissa ran into the tiny kitchen area and grabbed a steak knife. "Don't you ever punch me again, you shit!" she shrieked.

"You're nothing but a slut and you need to learn who's the boss around here."

Crouched, waving the knife, Melissa looked at John. "Don't come any closer." As she watched, an angry smile changed John's face into something horrible, and Melissa realized that this had gone much too far. "Calm down, baby," she said, straightening. "It's okay now. We can talk about this." Although she willed her body to relax, she kept the knife handy. This was a John she didn't know and didn't trust.

Slowly John walked toward her. "You gotta learn some respect for your husband."

"Don't, John baby," Melissa said, her voice now a whine.

"Yeah. Some respect."

Later, as she tried to tell the authorities exactly what happened next, she said that she didn't know. Exactly who moved first and how was a blank. She said she recalled nothing except John on the floor, blood seeping from his chest, the bloody knife still in her hand.

* * *

The phone rang and, as I reached for it, Ed swung his feet to the floor. "What have we got?" I asked the police dispatcher. When you're on overnight ambulance duty, you forget amenities like "Hello."

"Stabbing at 146 Colonial. Fred Stevens will pick up the rig and meet you at the scene. Don't go in until I clear you. We don't know exactly who did the stabbing and where the perp is."

"We're on our way." As I dressed I filled Ed in. It was only six minutes from the time we got the call until we pulled up in front of the Colonial Street address. Four police cars and the ambulance were already parked outside. Fred Stevens walked up to the car as Ed and I got out. "The cops say we can go in in about a minute," he told us.

"What's the story?"

"Domestic. From what I understand *she* stabbed *him*. He's bloody and in bad shape and she's hysterical, still holding the knife. As soon as they talk her down, we can go in."

"Okay, you guys," Merve Berkowitz yelled. "We're clear in here."

"Joan, you're listed as crew chief tonight. I'll get the stretcher." Fred handed the megaduffel to Ed.

As we walked quickly up the driveway, Ed said, "Fred is always somewhere else when things get messy."

"Yeah." I nodded, pulling on a second pair of latex gloves over the ones I already had on. If there was going to be lots of blood, I wanted extra protection. We ran in through the now-open front door and were directed to the kitchen. "The wife's outside," Eileen Flynn said. "She's in 308, hysterical. She's screaming, 'I love him. Don't let him die.' But she's the one who stabbed him. Go figure."

I knelt beside the body of a man in his mid-twenties. The bloodstain on the front of his blue linen shirt was about the size of my hand. He was pale and diaphoretic, and he was moaning quietly. Without my having to ask, Ed handed me a pair of heavy shears. I quickly cut up the front of the shirt, noticing that his breathing was shallow and rapid. I exposed his almost-hairless chest and saw that the area was bloody. I could see an open wound about two inches long, between two ribs just below his left nipple.

"Oxygen quick," I said. "And someone get a set of vitals." I grabbed the man's wrist and felt for a radial pulse. Although I moved my fingers several times, I found no beating. I reached for his carotid and found it, weak and fast but palpable. The presence of a carotid pulse and lack of a radial meant that he probably had a systolic blood pressure of between 60 and 80.

Ed opened the man's mouth and shook his head. Nothing blocking the airway. As Officer Flynn put a non-rebreather face mask over the man's nose and mouth, I watched his breathing more carefully—fast and shallow, about twice my rate. I ran my hands carefully over his ribs, then slipped my fingers underneath his chest, pulling them out repeatedly to look for fresh blood from an exit wound I might not be able to see. Fortunately I found none. "His ribs feel intact and I find no blood from his back," I said, partly to keep Ed apprised and partly to voice my findings so I'd remember them later.

"His breathing's lousy," Ed said, fastening the mask over the man's nose and mouth. "The wound's sucking."

Every breath our patient took was being pulled into his

chest cavity through the open stab wound. That air was filling what was ordinarily a vacuum and preventing the man's lungs from inflating properly. We needed to seal the injury. I placed my gloved palm over the wound and pressed. Fortunately Ed and I have worked together for so long that we usually can anticipate each other's needs, so he was already pulling a large trauma dressing from its heavy plastic envelope.

"Eileen," I said, "get me a kitchen towel."

Eileen quickly located a blue-and-white striped towel and started to hand it to me.

I knew she was really great in a medical emergency and she could function as part of our team. "Are you gloved?" I asked, reluctant to take my eyes off the man's chest and his respirations, which seemed a bit improved. When she said yes, I said, "Will you clean him off as best you can? I can't move my hand."

Carefully Eileen wiped the blood and sweat off the man's chest, making a dry place for us to tape a dressing. Meanwhile I knew Ed was cutting a good-size square of plastic from the packaging material of the dressing and finding wide adhesive tape. "I'm ready here," he said as Eileen enlarged the clean area.

"Great," I said. "Give me the patch." I took the plastic square and lifted my palm. Eileen wiped up the blood, still slowly flowing from the site, and I quickly placed the plastic over the wound. Holding it there with my palm, I watched Ed tape it down. He applied wide adhesive to the four sides, but left one corner untaped. Like a flutter valve, the open corner would allow air to escape when the patient exhaled and lessen the air pressure inside his chest that was keeping his lungs from expanding properly. When the man inhaled, the plastic would press tightly against his skin and prevent air from entering his chest cavity.

"Anyone know his name?" I asked.

"John Kirkwood," someone said.

"John," I said loudly, now able to move from his chest. "Can you hear me?" I got no response. I leaned closer to his ear. "John. Can you open your eyes?" Still no response. As I spoke I used my hands to check his head and neck for other injuries.

"Joan," Ed said. "I've got 75 over maybe 45 and a pulse of 110. Respirations are 34 and shallow." His breathing was too fast to be doing any good.

"Okay." I rubbed the knuckle of my index finger hard over John's breastbone and he moaned. "He reacts to pain." We needed to force oxygen deeper into his lungs. "Eileen, can you bag him for me and can you come with us? I really need an extra pair of hands."

"Sure," she said. Fred switched the oxygen tubing from the non-rebreather to the bag-valve mask and handed her the device. Eileen fitted the mask part over John's face, tipped his head to open his airway, and squeezed the bag, forcing pure oxygen into his lungs. "Do we have a stretcher and a longboard?"

"Right here," Fred said. "We're ready whenever you say."

"Let's get him out of here. We'll put the MAST on in the rig." Ed and Fred cut off the remainder of John's clothes. Now the MAST could be applied effectively.

Using a few of the police officers, we quickly logrolled John onto his side and I checked his back again. No wound. While we rolled him onto the long backboard, strapped him down, and lifted him onto the stretcher, Eileen never missed a beat. Ed strapped the oxygen tank to the foot of the stretcher and we quickly wheeled it to the rig. With the many hands we had, lifting him into the ambulance was easy. I looked at the collection of officers. "Will someone call the hospital and let them know we're coming? We're going to be real busy back there."

"Sure," Merve said. I saw that his eyes were still large. He was not used to dealing with violent crime.

I told Fred to go as soon as he was ready. During the six-minute drive to FGH, we awkwardly maneuvered the unconscious man into the MAST trousers, a device that looks like a very baggy pair of pants. When inflated, the MAST would increase his blood pressure and, theoretically, his chances for survival. I also checked his pulses and level of consciousness several times, noting that there was no change.

As we were about to inflate the MAST, Fred yelled that we were pulling into the ambulance bay. "This can wait," I said.

As the rig stopped, Ed and I jumped out and, with Fred's help, took out the stretcher while Eileen still calmly squeezed the bag of the BVM. As we entered the emergency room, several people directed us to trauma bay 1. There several gloved-and-ready nurses, doctors, and ancillary personnel were ready to receive him.

"Okay, guys," Dr. Morrison said, "what's the story?"

"Male, mid-twenties," I said. "Two-inch stab wound below his left nipple. Unable to determine how deep but there's no exit wound. Some blood, his shirt was stained about the size of my hand, but there's been little bleeding since we exposed the area. It was a sucking wound so we used an occlusive dressing. I think his breathing eased somewhat but we've been bagging him all the time.

Responsive only to pain. Last vitals were 78 over 40, 104 and 30 and shallow."

I watched as the team took over. While one nurse started bagging, others drew blood specimens, inserted IV lines, and hooked him to the machine that would automatically take vitals.

"Nice job, guys," Dr. Morrison said.

"Thanks," I said, catching my breath. "And thanks, Eileen. Nice work."

She beamed. "Always glad to help. I get little enough chance to use all this EMT training."

"Well, I'm always glad you're around," Ed said and Fred nodded.

The four of us cleaned up, changed the linen on the stretcher, and filled out the state paperwork. Eileen called headquarters and got additional information about the patient for us and for the hospital.

Just before we left, I asked Dr. Morrison, "How's he doing?"

"He'll make it. He's got a collapsed left lung but the knife missed the heart and most of the other vital organs so he's lucky. He'll be here for a while, but he'll live to fight again."

"Swell," I said dryly.

"How about the wife?" I asked Eileen.

"She's under arrest. It'll be up to the D.A."

I just shook my head and we walked out of the emergency room.

Bill Brown had worked at the A Plus Minimart for several months. Since he worked nights driving a newspaper delivery truck, this was a perfect way to increase his income. So from midnight to 6 or 7 A.M. he delivered papers, then he left that job and went directly to the minimart. There he took cash, helped with the gas pumps, and showed people how to use the microwave to heat their muffins and bagels until 2 P.M., when he finally went home to bed. It was a tough grind but he had money jingling in his jeans and the weekends off to spend it.

At the minimart things were very busy with morning commuters until about 10 A.M., then everything quieted down until lunchtime. Occasionally there was even time for Bill to relax and read a magazine from the rack. One Thursday morning in midsummer, Bill was sitting behind the counter reading the latest issue of *Sports Illustrated*. He looked up when a couple entered the store and glanced around, seemingly watching for people rather than for items to buy. Bill felt a bit uneasy but, since they seemed harmless, he looked back down at a photograph of Pete Sampras.

Suddenly a voice said softly, "Just take all the cash out of the register and put it in here." Then a small green sports bag was thrust in his face. He barely saw the bag, his gaze focused instead on the gun in the man's hand. He glanced at the woman who stood right behind and saw a gun in her hand as well.

Shit, he thought. Things like this don't happen in small suburban towns. He quickly opened the register, grabbed all the bills, and stuffed them into the bag. As the woman looked around, her eyes darting from the door to Bill, the man snatched the bag and, waving the gun, said, "Don't use the phone to call the cops."

Call the cops, Bill thought. Right. He watched the two walk quickly to their car and speed away. "Recent-model black Honda Civic," Bill said aloud over and over as he dashed for the door. He watched the back of the retreating vehicle and stared at the license plate. All he could make out was that it was a Florida plate with the letters HC at the end. "Like Honda Civic," he said. He ran back into the minimart and dialed 911.

Dispatcher Mark Thomas took the call and immediately pressed the radio call button. "GBY–639 to all cars in the field. Be on the lookout for a late-model Honda Civic, black, with Florida plates ending in the letters H-C. Unknown direction of travel from the A Plus Minimart. The occupants are said to be white, one male, one female. They are wanted in connection with a 10–14 that just occurred. If observed proceed with caution. Both suspects displayed weapons."

Will McAndrews listened to the notification and jotted the word Fla and the letters HC on the clipboard on the passenger seat of his patrol car. As he looked up, a black Honda was just passing him going south, toward the parkway. He peered at the license plate and, although he couldn't make out the letters, it looked like the Florida colors. He flipped on his lights and siren and pulled into traffic, watching cars part like the Red Sea in front of him. If the car he was pursuing wasn't the one involved in the robbery, then no harm would be done. It would just pull over and he'd check out the driver's license and registration and return to patrol.

But the Honda didn't pull over. Rather it picked up speed and began to weave around cars and vans, crossing a double yellow line and plunging forward. Will picked up his microphone. "Car 312 to 639 base. I am in pursuit of a black Honda Civic with Florida plates. Currently I'm southbound on Route 10, just passing the Red Foxx, doing about sixty."

"10–4, 312. 639 to all units. Car 312 is requesting backup, in pursuit of a 10–14 suspect. 317 and 318, 10–12 code 3. All other units clear this frequency."

As Will listened, both cars 317 and 318 called in that they were proceeding, lights and siren, to back him up. As the Honda turned onto Maple Avenue, he keyed the mike again. "Suspect vehicle just turned westbound onto Maple."

After the dispatcher relayed the new direction of travel, the airwaves were silent and the wail of the siren seemed unusually loud in Will's police car. When Will joined the Fairfax Police Department, he had been anxious for "real police work," high-speed chases, shoot-outs, and other forms of mayhem. Now, having been a member of the department for twelve years and having experienced very little of that type of drama, he wasn't sure he really wanted to.

The Honda was about five hundred yards in front of him and he lost sight of it momentarily as it turned a corner. "Suspect vehicle has now turned north on Chestnut," and a moment later, "Now he's going east on Lawrence, probably heading back to Route 10." He sped around the corner and followed the speeding Honda until it turned back onto Route 10. "He's on 10 now heading south again, probably toward the parkway." We could lose him if he gets onto the parkway, Will thought, worried.

"Will, this is 317." He recognized Merve Berkowitz's voice. "I'm on Main and he just flew by me." Will became aware of another police car just in front of him.

"305, this is 318. I'm at Maple and Willow, fifteen seconds behind you." Eileen Flynn was joining the chase.

Merve was now between Will and the Honda, and cars were pulling over to the side to let the high-speed procession pass. Just as the Honda neared the parkway entrance, Will watched as it suddenly fishtailed, spun around, and crashed into a telephone pole. As he and Merve pulled to a stop, both front doors of the Honda flew open and the occupants fled on foot in opposite directions. "I'll take him," Merve called, pointing to the tall, lanky man, now running across Route 10, dodging cars. "You get her." Almost simultaneously, the two men yelled, "Stop. Police officers." Their words had no effect on the fleeing figures.

As Will chased the woman who had scampered out of the passenger door, Merve took off after the driver, crossing Route 10 and running through the A&P parking lot. As he ran, Will saw the two men heading for a wooded area behind the supermarket.

Ahead of Will, the woman rushed down Route 10, then turned and ran around the back of Nick's Beer and Soda. "I'm getting too old for this," Will grumbled to himself as he began to puff. The woman was slowing and the distance between them was closing. She looked back and, seeing Will approaching, picked up a bit of speed, but Will pursued. As he got almost close enough to grab her, she suddenly collapsed in a heap and a small handgun skittered across the ground.

Using correct police procedure, Will stopped about five feet from the woman. "Put your hands out where I can see them." She didn't move. "I have a gun and I want to see your hands." When she still didn't move, he yelled, "Now!"

He approached the prone figure carefully, grabbed the woman's limp wrists, and handcuffed them behind her. He holstered his weapon. "You're under arrest," he panted, palms on his knees, trying to catch his breath. As he started to read her her rights, he noticed that she still hadn't reacted to anything he had done. Looking at her face, he saw that her eyes were closed and there was no movement. "Shit," he muttered. "The accident." Must be some kind of delayed injury. He grabbed his portable radio from his belt. "Portable 312 to GBY–639. I need an ambulance at this location for the female passenger from the car. She's under arrest, but she seems to be unconscious."

"10–4, 312, I'll notify FVAC."

I was at home and had been listening to the car chase on my scanner. It had sounded like something out of a TV cop show rather than a local incident, and the entire episode had taken on a surreal quality. I was now curious to see the outcome. When no one at headquarters answered the first call for the ambulance, I dialed police headquarters. "Fairfax Police, Mark Thomas."

"It's Joan, Mark. I've been listening to the whole thing on my scanner. I think there's no crew at headquarters, so I'll respond to the scene as the EMT. Hit the tones for a driver and an attendant."

"Thanks, Joan."

"Is everything under control there?" I asked.

"Yup. One under arrest but she's now unconscious, probably from when the get-away car hit a pole. They're behind Nick's."

As I strode to my car I heard Mark toning out for the rest of the crew.

I arrived at Nick's Beer and Soda, parked, and walked around to the rear. I pulled on a pair of latex gloves as I took in the scene quickly. Eileen Flynn and Will McAndrews were standing over the figure of a woman lying on the ground with her hands cuffed behind her. She was unkempt with straggly brown hair that looked like it hadn't been washed in a while, a red T-shirt, worn jeans, socks, and sneakers.

"Hi, Joan," Will said. "She's all yours. Her car hit a telephone pole about ten minutes ago, but from the way she was running, I think it might all be bullshit."

I bent over the seemingly unconscious woman. Her eyes were closed and her breathing was accelerated from her exertion, but even. I checked her carotid pulse and found it rapid but steady and strong, normal for someone who had just been running. "Hello," I said loudly, "can you hear me? Can you tell me your name?"

I got no response. I asked again and again got no answer, but I noticed that her eyelids were blinking. I shook my head and said, "I guess we'll do a full immobilization, but I think she's holding her eyes closed."

Will leaned over the prone woman. "Listen, lady," he said in a growl to her. "If you don't open your eyes right now, I'm going to have this paramedic here put the biggest needle she's got into you."

I'm not a paramedic and I have no needles of any kind, but she didn't know that and if it worked, so much the better.

Suddenly the woman's eyes flickered open. "Where am I?" She moaned theatrically.

Okay, I thought. Will's right. She's unconscious like I'm the tooth fairy.

"You're under arrest, lady," Eileen said. As Eileen read the woman her rights, I palpated her head, neck, back, arms, and legs to check for any tenderness or swelling. I felt nothing unusual, though I did notice a small abrasion on her forehead. When Eileen finished, I said, "Okay, tell me what hurts."

"My neck and back. My head hurts real bad."

"Were you wearing a seat belt?"

"Yeah, sure. I was wearing a seat belt. Wouldn't want to get a ticket, would I?" She glared at me.

I realized I was probably asking inane questions, but what else could I do? I needed whatever information I could get. "What's your name?" She continued to glare at me. "Mine's Joan, and since we're stuck with each other we might as well make the best of this."

"Trish," she said.

"Good, Trish. Where's the worst pain?"

As she considered her answer I heard the rig pull into the parking lot. "45–01 is on location." I recognized Steve Nesbitt's voice. I keyed the microphone on my portable. "45–24 to –01. We need to do a full immobilization and, whenever you're ready, we'll need the stretcher too."

"10–4, –24."

"Will, I'll need some help here."

"Officer Flynn's going to take care of her." To avoid charges of anything sexual, I guessed.

"Okay," I said as Eileen knelt beside the prone woman, pulled on a pair of latex gloves, and carefully held Trish's head to stabilize it. "We're going to have to turn her over carefully, to protect her neck. Then we'll collar her and roll her onto a board." I pointedly looked at the handcuffs holding Trish's hands behind her back. "We can't turn her over with those cuffs on."

Eileen nodded and spoke to the prisoner. "Listen, Trish," she said, "we're going to have to turn you over, and it will be very uncomfortable for you if we have to leave your hands behind your back. Will you behave, or do we have to do this the hard way?" The woman said nothing. "Trish," Eileen said firmly, "answer so we don't have to be here all day." Eileen is small, redheaded, and very attractive. However, when she gets tough, she's a force to be reckoned with. "Trish, don't make me ask again."

"All right," she grumbled.

Steve and Jill Tremonte arrived with the equipment. We quickly fastened a collar around Trish's neck and, while we all held on to our patient, Eileen unfastened the handcuffs. With Jill holding head stabilization, Eileen, Will, Steve, and I rolled the woman carefully onto a long backboard. Then Eileen used her cuffs and Will's to fasten Trish's wrists to the board's handholds. We strapped her down tightly to protect her neck and back, then lifted her onto the stretcher and strapped it down. If she had any idea of trying to get away, we weren't giving her any chance.

I noticed that Trish's lower abdomen bulged a bit. "Trish," I said, "are you pregnant?"

"About five months," she said, and started to cry. "That's why we did it. We have no money for the baby. That's why we did it."

Will and Eileen exchanged looks. She had just confessed to whatever the crime had been, but undoubtedly they would question her more thoroughly at the hospital, where they could get a formal statement. I was amazed that not once since the accident had Trish expressed any concern for the baby or for the man who had been in the car with her. I shrugged and we transported her to the hospital without incident, Eileen following in her patrol car.

While I was filling out the paperwork at Fairfax General, 45–02 arrived with the other robbery suspect, who was also immobilized and handcuffed. "Wow," I said to Merve as he followed the stretcher into an ER cubicle. "Crime and violence in Fairfax."

"Yeah," Merve said, looking down at a large tear in the knee of his uniform pants. "Crime, violence, and these pants were only a week old."

There was a long article about the "serious crime" in the local weekly paper the following Thursday, but it said little that I didn't already know. The following week there was no follow-up, and the lead story was about the town's efforts to trim the local school budget. Crime and violence doesn't sell papers in Fairfax.

Sometimes cops think of things that we, as focused EMTs, don't consider.

Marty Nobel was basically an indoor person. Actually, to be more accurate, he was a couch potato. He loved his TV, especially his collection of old black-and-white films. Recently retired, he now had the time that he had always wanted to watch his movies. He had set aside the month of August to create a filing system for his treasures. He used his son's old computer and a spreadsheet program to list his films, with director, major stars, year of release, and other pertinent data so he could sort on any category. With a library of over four hundred movies, it was a time-consuming job, and he loved it.

One morning he realized that he was out of floppy disks for backups. "Hon," he called to his wife of thirty-two years, "I'm heading to Staples. You need anything?"

"No, dear," she said, barely looking up from her morning's attack on the local newspaper's crossword puzzle. "Drive safe."

"Bye," he called, and walked outside. It was a wonderful August morning, unusually dry for this humid area. Marty closed his eyes and took a deep breath of suburban summer. "Nice," he said aloud. After a few moments of enjoying the day, he walked toward his car. As he passed one of his wife's prized rosebushes, he leaned over to see how the flowers smelled.

Suddenly his hand was on fire. He looked down at the bumblebee, now unable to remove its stinger from his right palm. With already-shaking hands, Marty swatted at the bug until the dead body fell to the ground. "Damn," he muttered. Then his heart began to pound, and he sprinted for his front door. As he ran, his breathing thickened and he began to feel faint. Sweat tickled his armpits and ran down his chest. Light-headed and dizzy, he made it to the concrete slab at the base of his front steps before he became too weak to go any farther. "Anne," he yelled, holding on to the iron stair railing. "Anne, help."

Almost immediately the front door opened. "What happened?" Anne cried. "Marty. What's wrong?"

"Some little bastard ... stung me ..." He puffed, having difficulty getting his breath. His hand was on fire, his tongue and throat felt swollen, and he was becoming too weak to stand.

"I'll call an ambulance," Anne said, dashing back into the house.

As Marty watched her disappear through the front door, he collapsed, hitting his face on the concrete step.

"Fairfax Police to Fairfax Ambulance."

Heather Franks keyed the mike at headquarters as I stuffed the last bite of my doughnut into my mouth. I had been visiting with Heather and Tom after getting my mail and catching up on the announcements on the bulletin board. I try to do it once a week or so, but it usually happens only once a month. We had been chatting about how Heather and Tom, both school employees, were spending their summer.

"Base on."

"Respond to 1364 Oak Hill for a reaction to a bee sting. The name is Nobel. I talked to the wife and she's pretty hysterical."

"10–4," Heather said. "45–01 is responding to 1364 Oak Hill for a bee sting."

"Could be bullshit," Tom said. "Probably nothing."

"Yeah," Heather said. "Hey, Joan, we're alone. Come along?"

I had a zillion things to do, but I can't turn down a call. "Sure," I said, following the couple to the rig. Heather drove out of the garage and, after pressing the button to close the big garage doors, I jumped into the back while Tom got into the shotgun seat.

"If this is real," Tom said over the sound of the siren, "we could sure use a medic."

"If the town ever gets around to funding the program. . . ." It was a topic that had been going round and round for months. Reluctant to authorize the tax increase of about forty dollars per household that would be required to staff a fly car similar to Prescott's, the town had been waffling, establishing committees and ordering feasibility studies. The ambulance corps had been at the forefront of the drive to establish paramedic services, and we were all frustrated by how long it was taking to get the program going.

Silently the three of us drove through town toward Oak Hill, in the Floral Court development, watching the traffic pull to the side of the road to let us pass. Heather turned right onto Oak Hill and we checked the numbers on the mailboxes. "There it is," Tom said, pointing to a white mailbox. We pulled into the driveway and, gloved and ready for whatever we might find, we trotted to the open front door.

"Hello," Tom shouted. "Ambulance!"

"There's blood here on the step," I said. "Not a lot but it looks recent."

Heather walked into the front hall. "Ambulance!"

There was nothing but silence. "Heather, look around inside. Joan, let's try out back," Tom suggested. He went one way and I went the other around the building. When we saw each other again as we rounded the house, we shrugged. "There's a car in the garage. Did you find anything?"

"Not a thing," I said.

When we arrived back at the front door Tom yelled the same question to Heather, now in the front hall, having returned from the upstairs of the house. "I can't find anything," she called. "No patient, no blood, nothing."

At that moment police car 308 came to a stop behind the ambulance, and Stan Poritsky walked up to us. "What's up?"

Heather came out of the front door. "There's blood on the front step but we can't find anyone," she said. "Maybe we'd better get more manpower and start a search."

"Yeah," Tom said. "The car's here and God knows what kind of shape the victim might be in."

"Hang on," Stan said, grabbing the sector car cell phone. "Let me call FGH ER." He dialed quickly.

"Hello, this is Officer Poritsky from Fairfax Police. Did anyone come in within the last few minutes with a bee sting?"

There was a pause, then he said, "And the name?"

I could see his body relax. "Okay, thanks." He turned to us. "His wife drove him in."

"Lord," Tom said. "Didn't anyone have the good sense to call us off?"

"Relax, baby," Heather said, patting her husband's arm. "They had other things on their mind, and it probably never occurred to them."

I hung out with Tom and Heather and, just before noon, we had a call for a woman who had been attacked by a raccoon. Disbelieving, we drove to the scene to discover that, while walking with her boyfriend through a lightly wooded area, not only had she been attacked and chased by a large raccoon, but she had three long, deep lacerations on her leg. Ordinarily the injury wouldn't have required an ambulance, but we knew she would need rabies shots so we advised her to let us transport her so the hospital could begin dealings with the Health Department.

After we finished our paperwork and made up the stretcher, Heather, Tom, and I cornered Rosemary Harper, one of the ER nurses we knew well. It was relatively quiet so we asked her to tell us about our nonpatient.

"Actually he's lucky his wife did what she did. He almost died in the parking lot. When we got him in here he had no blood pressure. I mean, he was *out*. And he had a four-inch head lac that wouldn't stop bleeding." I love

ER nurse slang. Head lac, for head laceration. I guess every profession has its jargon.

"Phew. Did he know he was allergic?" I asked. "Didn't he have an epi stick?"

"He was stung twenty years ago and had a reaction. So the doctor warned him and gave him an epi pen. But when the wife looked for it this morning, she discovered that it was totally outdated. He had never thought to get the prescription refilled because he hadn't been stung so he hadn't used the old one."

We all shrugged. Epinephrine can save your life, but only if you have nonexpired medication ready for instant use. "Is he okay?"

"I think so. He's in trauma 1, feeling much better now. But it took almost three hours to get his blood pressure back up. Eventually he'll need stitches for his head too."

"Glad he didn't wait for us," Heather said.

"Yeah," Rosemary said. "I seldom see a case where leaving the scene is the right thing to do, but in this case it worked out fine."

"Occasionally it does," Tom said, wheeling the stretcher toward the door. We waved good-bye to our raccoon-injured patient and looked forward to lunch.

When I told this story to a group of other EMTs, one told about an even more bizarre call they had had.

"It was almost midnight and I was ready to get home when the klaxon sounded. We were dispatched to an address right around the corner from headquarters. On the way there, the 911 operator told us that she had been called by someone who said she was having a heart attack, then became silent. The line remained open and the dispatcher tried to get the woman back on the line, but she got no response.

"So we get onto the right street but everything's dark. I mean, dark as the inside of a cat. No house lights, no nothing.

"We use the spotlight to illuminate the mailboxes but half of them have no addresses and we've got no landmarks.

"So we drive around counting, trying to interpolate from the numbers we *did* have, to locate the right house. We finally agree that this one house has to be it so we pull into the driveway.

"We see that there's a light on at the back so we pound on the door. Nothing. We pound and yell. Still nothing.

" 'I'm for breaking down the goddamn door,' my buddy says.

" 'Me too,' I agree, but the crew chief won't do it. 'It's breaking and entering,' he says. 'We have no right to do that.'

" 'I don't give a flying fuck,' my buddy says. 'I'm getting the crowbar.'

"Fortunately, before my buddy and the crew chief come to blows, the cops arrive. They break a small pane of glass beside the front door and we're in. We find the poor woman on the floor in the back bedroom still clutching the phone. We did CPR and got her to FGH stat, but the story, I'm sorry to say, doesn't have a happy ending. We couldn't revive her.

"The doctors assured us that the delay in getting to her had no effect, that her heart attack had been so massive that nothing could have revived her. But . . . it's a hard decision to violate a law to try to save a life. I'm for breaking and entering every time."

Another EMT who was also a firefighter added another short story.

"About three years ago we got a fire call and arrived at the house. It was the right one and everything, and we can hear the alarm sounding inside. We pound but over the sound of the alarm no one can hear a thing. We pound some more, still nothing. So we do what we have to and break down the door.

"There's a man standing in the front hall, fanning the smoke alarm with a newspaper. 'Who called us?' one of our guys asks when the alarm finally stops. 'I don't have the faintest,' the homeowner says. 'Got an alarm system?' someone asks. 'No,' he says.

"So eventually we come to discover that the call was deliberately made by a kid in an upstairs bedroom when his father burned the steaks. The kid thought it was funny. The department paid for a new door and I think the kid's still grounded."

"Ain't teenagers great?" several people said at once.

We also work very closely with the fire department, both in Fairfax, where the two agencies are entirely separate, and in Prescott, where the rescue squad is part of the fire department.

It came in first as a fire call. I was in the ambulance and we were on the way back from FGH when we heard it. "Fairfax Fire Department to all responding men and apparatus. We have an automatic alarm at the Mercury Nursing Center on Barclay Street. Engines 44–31 and 44–33 are responding."

Automatic alarms are almost always false, but the fire

department dutifully responds to each as if it were the real thing. "Fairfax Fire Department to all units. We have an update. There is a confirmed fire in the recreation room. 45–01 respond for a possible injury."

"10–4," our driver, Dave Hancock, said into the mike. He efficiently flipped all the switches to turn on the flashing lights and the siren. "Guess it's a real one, Joan."

As we drove toward the nursing home, we heard various units call in. Chief Bradley called that he was 10–19, on location. Almost immediately he added, "44–11 to the rescue. Expedite."

"Shit," I muttered, reaching for a pair of gloves. "Sounds bad."

Marge Talbot nodded from the front seat as I handed her a pair of gloves. In only another minute we arrived in front of the nursing center. I climbed out and was quickly approached by Chief Bradley. "The fire's out but one of the residents is badly burned." He pointed and I sprinted, followed by Marge. I knew Dave would be getting the equipment we would need.

As we ran, firefighters pointed the way, like the people in charge of big-city marathons, directing the runners through the various intersections. We arrived to find an older man on the floor, with several members of the nursing staff pouring water over him. The room was filled with smoke and the smell of burned flesh.

"What happened?" I asked.

"Cigarette. It ignited his shirt. We used the fire blanket but it seemed to do no good. His pants seem to have protected his lower body, but he's burned badly from the waist up."

I knelt beside the frail-looking man and took his hand. "We're here now," I said. "Just try to relax."

"Not so bad," he said, squeezing my hand in a surprisingly strong grip.

I looked him over. He had what looked like second- and third-degree burns over much of his upper body and arms. Miraculously his face was uninjured. "Easy with the water," I said, seeing that the man was shivering. "We need the big water-gel blanket."

"And the Reeves," Marge added.

Water-gel is wonderful stuff. Sheets of heavy gauze-like material are impregnated with a substance that's a bactericide, a cooling agent, and a mild anesthetic. It cools the burns, kills germs, and makes the patient more comfortable all at the same time.

Marge, on the gentleman's other side, gently took his wrist in an unburned area and checked his pulse. "He's got a weak radial pulse," she said, "at about 90." She yelled to Dave, "Set up the oxygen."

As Dave retrieved a non-rebreather mask, several firemen arrived and opened the Reeves stretcher and a sheet of water-gel. "We have to be careful with hypothermia," I said to Marge.

One of the workers leaned over and said, "He's blind. I just thought you should know."

"Thanks," I said.

"I'm scared," the man said softly.

"I know, but I'm holding your hand and I won't let go." The noise level was rising as the firefighters used large fans to clear the light pall of smoke from the room and others spread the water-gel blanket over the Reeves. Several firefighters were yelling instructions to others.

"Hey," I called out. "Can you keep the noise down a bit! I can't talk to the patient."

Everyone looked around at everyone else, but the

noise level dropped considerably. "Can you tell me your name?" I asked.

"Cliff Politis," the man said, his voice firm.

"Cliff, what happened?"

He looked at me with sightless eyes. "It was only one cigarette. They don't let me smoke, but I have so little else. So I snuck into the corner by the window. But it fell. On my shirt, I think."

"Where was he when this happened?" I asked one of the aides.

"In his wheelchair over there," she said, pointing to a dripping, smoke-stained wheelchair.

I spotted a green oxygen cylinder attached to the back and saw a nasal canula dangling over one arm. "Was he on oxygen?"

"Yes," Cliff said softly. He squeezed my hand. "I usually turn it off, but I guess I forgot."

I just shook my head. Probably he had been using the canula, so his clothing had become impregnated with extra oxygen. When he dropped the cigarette it flared and, when the attendants threw the fire-retardant blanket over him, it trapped the flames, with the canula still pumping oxygen and feeding the fire, against his body.

The smell was overpowering, a combination of charred clothing and burned meat. It's an odor that, once smelled, is never forgotten.

One fireman arrived with a second burn sheet and we spread it over the man's upper body and arms. "Get a regular blanket for his lower body," I said. "He's getting really cold."

Pete Williamson arrived in the room at his efficient but seemingly unhurried pace. He's a paramedic in the city, and, though he cannot function as one with FVAC since we're only authorized to perform basic life support, his experience and calm, unflappable attitude are always an asset. Together we rolled Cliff onto his side and I quickly checked his back. It was seriously burned from neck to waist. We rolled him onto the water gel–covered Reeves and made him as comfortable as we could. All the while the man kept a tight grip on my hand.

Pete looked at me. "I think we might take that top burn-sheet off. He's probably getting hypothermic."

"Good idea," I said. We removed the wet sheet, carefully wiped the unburned parts of Cliff's body, and covered him with sterile burn dressings.

Marge told me the rough vitals she had obtained as Dave put the non-rebreather mask over Cliff's mouth and nose.

"Any idea how much area is burned?" Pete asked.

"Upper back, chest, and both arms," I answered. "About 36 percent." I used the rule of nines to estimate the percent of burned area. To do that we divide the body into eleven areas, then count 9 percent of the body for each. Cliff got one "nine" for his upper back, one for his upper chest, and one for each arm—four nines equal 36 percent of his body burned, and it was mostly third degree. The fact he had mostly third-degree burns accounted for his lack of pain. In third-degree, or full-thickness, burns, the underlying nerve tissue is damaged and its ability to send pain messages is compromised. Thus, although a third-degree burn is more serious than a second-degree, or partial-thickness burn, the amount of pain is often less.

By now four firefighters had already used the Reeves' handles to lift Cliff onto the stretcher and were wheeling the stretcher toward the rig as I ran alongside, clinging to the injured man's hand. Quickly Marge, Pete, and Dave gathered our equipment and followed. A nursing home attendant stuffed some papers into my hand. "That's his information," she said. "It's got everything you'll need, I think." I glanced at the papers and found that I could avoid asking Cliff a battery of questions. I looked at his date of birth. Cliff was eighty-six. And he was a diabetic, which probably accounted for his blindness.

Marge and Pete climbed in beside me and Dave got behind the wheel. "Where to?" Dave yelled.

"To the trauma center, and let's not waste time."

"Will do," Dave said, and he started toward St. Luke's Trauma Center's ER. Eventually Cliff would be transferred to the center's new burn unit.

I held Cliff's hand while Pete and Marge adjusted the oxygen, took vitals, and further bandaged his burned arms. "You won't let go, young lady?"

"Young lady?" I smiled. "If you're talking to me, let me thank you from the bottom of my heart. I'm gray-haired and a grandmother."

"When you're eighty-six, any woman still alive is a young lady."

We all laughed, marveling at the man's sense of humor in this terrible situation.

In a few minutes we arrived at the trauma center and Cliff was quickly transferred to their gurney. At least six people hovered around him, one just holding his hand and talking softly to him. I felt a bit bereft. For a while I had been important to him, if only as a hand to hold.

I was saddened to read in the local paper that Cliff survived for only five days before succumbing to his injuries. I knew that the combination of serious burns, his age, and his generally debilitated condition decreased his chances, but still I had hoped. I hope with every patient, and most of the time things go well.

No matter how long a person is an EMT, there are always new situations and unexpected consequences.

It was a hot midsummer morning, and Ed and I responded to a report of an accident on the parkway north of Route 10. It was a difficult spot to get to since that section of the parkway has two narrow lanes in each direction, with no shoulder. Heavy woods border the roadway. Whenever there is a bad accident, the traffic behind it backs up quickly and the traffic in the opposite direction slows to a crawl with rubberneckers. This morning was no different.

Ed and I had called in that we were responding. We hoped that we could get to the scene by going to the exit immediately north of Route 10 and heading south. We hadn't reckoned on the fire engines that now blocked the southbound lane as well. Traffic was at a complete standstill. We managed to get to a slightly widened area and pulled off the road about a quarter of a mile from the scene. From there we walked.

By the time we arrived at the scene I was breathless and covered with sweat, but there was work to do. An older-model van was overturned and resting on the driver's side. We could see the driver inside, lying on the driver's door. Linda Potemski and Nick Abrams were leaning in through the shattered windshield, talking to the man.

"What can we do to help?" I asked Nick.

He stood up. "The guy's arm is trapped beneath the

van," he said. "The fire department is getting ready to try to lift it with air bags so we can get him out. And the helicopter's in the air, landing at the high school."

I contemplated the problem. Several firefighters were using heavy rope to tie the van to the front bumper of engine 44–31, now totally blocking the southbound lane. A second rope was being tied around a large tree so that, once tight, the two ropes would keep the van from shifting. Others were using a stair-step arrangement of two-by-fours to further steady the vehicle.

While Linda stayed with the driver, Ed, Nick, and I stood and watched. "I'd love for one of you to get inside," Nick said, "but not while they're fooling with the air bags." Someone handed Linda, a small woman to begin with, a heavy fire helmet, which nearly tipped her over. "For protection while we're working," he told her.

Finally several firemen slid two eighteen-inch-square air bags, sandwiched between flat pieces of wood to avoid possible puncture, beneath the driver's side of the van. The heavy rubberized devices were attached to the pressure regulator of a Scott air pack.

"Okay," Chief Bradley yelled, "listen only to me."

The area became silent. To avoid any potentially dangerous confusion, one person, usually the senior fire officer, would be in charge of raising the van. "Up on red," he said, and the fireman working the pressure valve set it to begin to inflate the red air bag. "Stop," he said. "Now up on yellow."

Slowly, with alternate increases of the inflation of the red and yellow bags, the van lifted. As it did so, the stair-step chocks were slid deeper beneath the van, further stabilizing it. Finally we could look beneath the driver's door and see the man's arm, which was in remarkably good shape.

"Okay," Chief Bradley said. "I think that's got it."

Several firemen looked under the door and agreed that the man's arm was now free. Nick, Ed, and I walked over to Linda. "What do you need?" I asked.

"I think we can get a collar on him now."

"I'll get the collar bag and set up the longboard and such," Nick said.

"Ed, can you get inside?" Linda asked. "I don't know anything about the rest of the guy's body."

While Ed got a helmet, I crouched with Linda. "How is he?"

"He seems really good," she said. "His vitals are fine and he's been talking to me all along. He says his arm hurts, but not too badly. I don't know whether this is really a chopper job, but from the mechanism of injury, I figured it was the best bet."

"He's amazingly lucky," I said. I handed Linda the regular-size collar she requested and together we fastened it around the driver's neck.

"My back's killing me," Linda said when she finished. "Can you take over head stabilization?"

"Sure," I said, and we quickly switched places. Linda straightened, rubbed her back, then plunked the heavy helmet on my head.

I looked over my patient who appeared to be about sixty with a ruddy complexion. He was seemingly unaffected by his accident. "What's your name?" I asked.

"Miguel," he said.

"Nice to meet you," I said. "I'm Joan. And I wish we had met under better circumstances. Can you move that arm?"

"I'm stuck on something," he said.

"Okay. We'll find out what and get you out of here. Can you wiggle your fingers?"

"Yeah. But my shoulder and upper arm really burn."

"I'll bet. Ed's down there checking out the rest of your body. How do you feel?"

"My chest hurts a little. Get me out of here, okay?"

"As quickly as we can." I saw Ed climbing around inside the van checking the man's legs. When he held one of Miguel's shoes, I said, "Ed's near your feet. Can you wiggle your toes?"

"Sure," Miguel said. Ed nodded and together we checked the other foot.

"That's great," he yelled. "Everything seems clear down here."

Several firefighters poked and snooped, unable to ascertain why we couldn't get Miguel free. "His shoulder's jammed," one said. "I think we'll need the jaws."

"We can't cut the posts," another said, "because the lower A-post is the only thing holding the car together. It'll collapse on him if we cut it."

"Don't let them do that!" Miguel yelled.

"Don't worry, they're the greatest and they know just what to do. They'll explore every option and pick the best one."

"Are you sure?" he asked.

"I'm here with you," I said, "and I'm not leaving. And I'm not going to let them do anything to hurt either one of us."

Finally, after a lot of discussion and mind changes, they finally agreed on the air chisel. I found it interesting to listen to them discussing options the same way several

EMTs do at an accident scene. Fortunately everyone's a team player.

"Miguel," I said, "they're going to use a very loud piece of equipment to get you out of here. It'll be tough on the ears but it's the best way."

"If you say so. Just get me out of here. My shoulder's starting to really hurt."

The air chisel is the noisiest piece of equipment in the fire department's arsenal. It bangs on the metal, cutting it slowly.

"Hang on, everyone," Chief Bradley said. "Here we go."

The noise was almost deafening but we all had no choice but to endure. I tried to hold Miguel's head as still as I could while the chisel cut across the roof of the car about two feet behind the windshield then toward the front on both sides, opening the roof like a flap.

Finally Miguel was free. Awkwardly, with Linda and Nick holding his shoulders and Ed pushing on his legs and hips, we got him onto a long backboard and onto the stretcher.

Linda examined the man's arm and found a large road rash on his shoulder. There was some pain when she touched it, but his pulse and neurological function were fine.

We quickly put oxygen on him and drove him the short distance to the helicopter, where the flight nurses were waiting. They quickly got an IV line started and him inside.

"Lucky guy," Linda said as the helicopter prepared to lift off. "He seems to have gotten out of this real easy."

"Seems to have."

                              *   *   *

The monthly meeting of Fairfax VAC was held the following week, and, as Ed and I walked in, Linda found me. "Remember that guy from last week?"

"Sure. Why?"

"I ran into one of the flight nurses. He had a crushed shoulder and every left side rib was separated from his spine. Every one. Most of them were separated at the front too, and his sternum was fractured."

"You're kidding," I said.

"Not only that, but he had a bruised heart and two bruised kidneys. Luckily nothing life threatening, so eventually he'll be okay, but I never expected so much damage from the way he was talking to us."

Ed and I shook our heads. It's amazing. We treat every patient for the worst case, even when we think it's minor. We treat strains and sprains as if they were fractures and assume that any head wound involves a brain injury. Most of the time when we think someone's badly hurt it turns out to be minor. This time we were all glad we had treated Miguel for the worst case, because it was.

Chapter 7

It was late afternoon on a rainy Sunday in May and I was just pulling into a parking space outside of the Fairfax A&P when the tones went off. "Fairfax Police to Fairfax Ambulance."

"Ambulance on," a voice said. I perked up my ears.

"The ambulance is needed on Hunter's Hill Road at the bad curve for a personal injury auto accident."

I groaned inwardly. That curve had been a terrible spot with at least one serious accident each month until about three years earlier, when the highway department put up flashing lights, large yellow arrows, and speed warning signs to alert drivers that the sharp curve turn heading outbound from town could not be taken safely at over twenty-five miles per hour. Since then the number of accidents had dropped but the ones that did occur were usually serious.

"10–4," Dave Hancock said from headquarters. "We've got a driver and an attendant in quarters. Can you please tone out for an EMT to meet us at the scene."

"Will do."

I was already grabbing my FVAC portable radio. "45–22 to FPD."

"Go ahead, Ed." Strangely enough, when it's a bad call

the dispatchers frequently lapse into informal radio communication, using first names instead of unit numbers.

"I'm at the Fairfax A&P, en route to the scene at the bad curve."

"10–4," the dispatcher said. As I started my car I heard him inform the rig that I was on the way. Since the accident scene was only a short distance away, I arrived well before the ambulance. I parked and quickly surveyed the damage to people and vehicles. A small black Toyota had been heading out of town and had tried to take the curve too quickly on the rain-slick road. It had hit an equally small beige Ford head on. There were several Fairfax police officers already at the scene, directing traffic and seeing to scene safety. Eileen Flynn approached me. "The woman in the Ford is out and walking around. She's complaining of a banged-up knee and some pain on her breastbone from the seat belt."

"And him?" I asked, gesturing toward the man still behind the wheel of the Toyota.

"He's more seriously hurt, I think," Eileen told me. "He's got chest and back pain and lots of pain in his left leg."

"Thanks, Eileen," I said. As I started toward the Toyota, I saw Heather Franks get out of her car and retrieve her crash kit from her trunk. "Tom's away," she said as she approached, referring to her husband who also rode with FVAC, "but I thought you might need extra hands. What can I do?"

"Glad to have you," I said. "If you can take care of the woman from the Ford, I'll work with the guy in the Toyota."

"Sure," Heather said, walking toward the woman who was now talking with Detective Irv Greenberg.

Confident that the woman was in good hands, I turned my attention to the man who was yelling in pain, still behind the wheel of the Toyota. As I approached the car I made a mental note of its condition for my report, and to assess the possibility of injuries to the driver. The car was totaled. The front end was crushed to about half its size but the windshield was intact. As I got to the driver's side door I noted that the steering wheel was also intact, not bent or compressed. Okay, I thought, his head didn't break the windshield and his chest didn't hit the steering wheel hard enough to break it. Knowing that stabilizing the man's head was the first priority, I said, "Sir, don't move your head. I'm going to get into the backseat and hold you but you must try not to move."

"Okay," he said. "But I hurt so much."

I carefully opened the back door and got into the car with as little movement of the vehicle as possible. I placed my gloved palms on either side of the man's head and said, "Sir, tell me where it hurts most."

"My leg and my back and my chest." Fear and anxiety colored every word.

"Okay, sir," I said, my voice deliberately pitched a bit lower and speaking especially clearly to penetrate his fear. "My name's Ed. What's yours?"

"My name's Norman Kobelev but everyone calls me Nomad."

"That's an odd name. Maybe you'll explain it to me later. Right now I want you to slow your breathing down and tell me what part of your back hurts."

"All over."

"That doesn't help me a lot. Is it mostly low, like in the small of your back, or higher up? Without moving, try to go over your body mentally and tell me."

"I guess it's around my chest."

"Good. Now take a deep breath for me and tell me whether it hurts more when you do that."

He took a slow deep breath. "No. Not too much more. It's just all around my ribs and chest. And my leg."

"Which leg hurts?"

"My left. I think it's broken."

"Can you wiggle the toes on that foot?"

He paused, then said, "Yes."

"That means there's good nerve function all the way down." I heard the siren on the approaching rig. "It sounds like the ambulance is here. We'll have you out of here in no time and on the way to the hospital." I wanted to keep his mind occupied so I continued to ask questions. "Do you remember the accident? Did you lose consciousness at all?"

"I remember. I guess I was going too fast and I lost control. The road's very slippery, you know. The rain and all."

I saw that his shoulder harness was still in place. "I see you have your seat belt on," I said.

"Well," he said, "not the lap part."

I looked at the shoulder harness. It was the automatic passive restraint kind that was in fashion for a few years before air bags became mandatory. "So the shoulder harness was across your chest but you had no lap belt. Did you slide down?"

"I guess. That's how I hurt my leg."

At that moment, Dave Hancock walked up to the driver's window. "What's the story, Ed?"

"He's complaining of front and back rib pain and pain in his left leg. Neuros seem okay on that side. He had a shoulder belt on but no lap belt so he did a down-and-under." The phrase down-and-under indicated that he had slid down the seat and under the dash before the shoulder harness stopped his progress.

Dave leaned in through the broken driver's window. "He's got a nasty laceration under his chin, Ed," he said, "probably from the shoulder belt. KED?"

"Can you check his leg first?"

Dave leaned into the car and ran his gloved hands over Nomad's left thigh. The man screamed when Dave touched anywhere between his knee and his waist. "I think his femur's broken," Dave said.

Oh, great, I thought. There's no room to splint it before we get him out of the car, and it's going to hurt like hell when we move it, unsplinted, out of the vehicle. Oh, well, I thought. We'll do the best we can.

I quickly considered whether doing a full, slow extrication was worth the time involved. In addition to his anxiety level, he was sweaty and his pulse was rapid. With a broken femur and possible damage to the femoral artery, I decided to do a rapid extrication. "Just get a collar and longboard," I said to Dave.

As Dave left to get the equipment we would need, I said, "We think your left thigh bone might be broken. We'll get you out of this car quickly, but it's going to hurt like crazy. We'll try our best to cause you as little pain as we can."

Through the front windshield I could see Heather, Irv Greenberg, and a bystander slowly lower the woman from the Ford to the ground, with a long backboard behind her. She would be ready to go long before we would, and I knew that Heather would take good care of her.

Dave returned with a collar and we quickly placed it

around Nomad's neck. "That hurts my neck," he yelled. "And it's pressing on my chest. I can't breathe."

"I'm sorry but this has to be," I said. "It's to protect you from further injury, and we can't take you out of here without it."

"But I can't breathe and my leg is killing me."

"Take a slow deep breath for me." When he did, I said, "That's good. Dave's got some oxygen for you to help your breathing. Do you have any ongoing medical problems?" Dave put a non-rebreather face mask over Nomad's nose and mouth so he would be breathing 100 percent oxygen.

"No."

"Do you take any medication on a regular basis?"

"Yes. For anxiety." He named a medication that was unfamiliar to me. I would write it down when we were on our way to the hospital. The patient's need for anxiety medication told me that it would be doubly important to keep him calm.

"Okay. Dave's got the long backboard. I want you to cross your hands on your belly and don't move them. You let us do all the work."

"Hi, guys," Tim Babbett said as he climbed into the front passenger seat.

"Hi, Tim," I said. "Nomad, this is Tim and he's going to help us get you out of here."

"Do it quick. I hurt everywhere."

Dave leaned in through the now-open driver's door. "I'll take charge of this leg. I've got several firemen"— he smiled—"I mean firefighters to help with the board."

I glanced out the front window and saw that several firefighters were spreading kitty litter all over the road surface to sop up the oil and gasoline that was leaking from both vehicles. Several more were supporting the longboard. Boy, I thought, it's nice to have lots of muscle in situations like this. "Nomad, we're going to turn you so your leg is out of the car then take you out feet first onto a board."

Dave slid the board onto the side of the seat and maneuvered it under Nomad's left buttock. Several burly firefighters held the free end of the board. "This is going to be the bad part," Dave said as he held Nomad's left leg.

"Let's do it," I said. "On my count. One, two, three." On "three" we turned our patient's body and Dave lifted his left leg. As the leg moved, Nomad screamed. When Tim seemed hesitant, I said, "Let's get this done." Dave got Nomad's leg on the board and we finished turning him, then, when I had transferred head stabilization to Tim, we slid him out. Only then did I discover that two more firefighters were holding a large yellow plastic sheet over the entire driver's side of the car to keep us dry. I looked at one, smiled, and said, "Thanks." While I got out of the back of the car, Dave and several others began to strap Nomad to the board. When his entire body was secure and his head was held tightly with yellow head blocks and lots of duct tape, they placed the board on the waiting stretcher.

At my instruction, Tim ran back to the rig and returned with a Sagar splint, a three-foot-long metal device that would immobilize Nomad's broken femur.

"We're going to put something on your leg," I explained while I loosened a few lower body straps and placed the shoulder of the device in Nomad's crotch. I smiled at him. "I know this feels weird but this device is going to pull on your leg and make some of the pain disappear."

"Are you sure you know what you're doing?" Nomad asked.

"You just wait," I said.

I hooked on the ankle strap and, when it was all in place, I extended the pole of the device until it was pulling hard, stretching Nomad's leg. "Does that help the pain?" I asked. A traction splint usually provides dramatic pain relief.

"Yes," Nomad said, "but my back and chest hurt. And this collar is killing me. And can you take this mask off my face?"

At least he's not complaining about his leg anymore, I thought.

As he finished bandaging the laceration under Nomad's chin, Dave looked into his eyes. "Just hang on a little longer," he said.

"I hope so. My chest and back hurt like hell."

We finished strapping Nomad to the board and then belted him to the stretcher. With the help of several firefighters, we lifted the stretcher into the ambulance. Heather was already inside with the woman from the Ford. I climbed in and Heather quickly filled me in on the woman's condition. There was little more wrong with her than I had been told when I arrived. "Do you need me?" Heather asked.

"Not really, if you need to go. I've got Tim to help back here and I think everyone's doing okay."

"Great. If you're sure."

"I'm sure."

Dave said, "Do you want to go to FGH or St. Luke's?"

"I think we're okay for Fairfax General." The patients were both stabilized, and I didn't think their injuries warranted the extra travel time that it would take to drive from this part of town to the trauma center. "Just give us a minute to get a quick set of vitals."

"Okay."

Tim took vitals on the woman, now fully immobilized on a longboard, while I checked Nomad's blood pressure, pulse, and respiration rate. I was glad to note that his vitals were all within normal limits and he was now tolerating the oxygen mask, although still complaining about it and everything else.

During our trip to Fairfax General Hospital, partly to keep them occupied, I gathered information from both patients for the PCRs. I was gratified to note that Nomad was still complaining about his back and chest, but not about his leg. The traction splint was obviously doing its job.

"You were going to tell me how you got the nickname Nomad," I said when, for the third time, he asked me to remove the oxygen mask and the hard cervical collar.

Around the mask he explained, "My little brother couldn't say Norman, so he started calling me Nomie. Nomie became Nomad and it just stuck."

When we arrived at FGH, we transferred care of our patients to the emergency room staff and, while Dave and Tim put clean linen on the stretcher and tidied up the back of the rig, I completed the paperwork on both patients.

"Hey, Ed," Dr. Morrison called. "You should see this." He led me over to a bank of X rays hanging on their lighted boxes. "See here?" he said, pointing to an area high up in Nomad's spine.

"Yeah," I said, not yet understanding exactly what I was looking at.

Dr. Morrison pointed to the spine. "Here. See the second cervical vertebra? It's broken clear through."

I gasped, stared, and understood. C2, it's called. And if the spinal cord is damaged at C2, the patient dies.

"Fortunately," Dr. Morrison said, "there was no displacement of the bones and the spinal cord is undamaged."

"Holy shit!" I exclaimed, realizing the impact of what he was saying. One wrong move during Nomad's extrication and the spinal injury would have killed him.

"Who was holding head stabilization?" Dr. Morrison asked.

"I was."

"Good job. Very good job."

"He wasn't complaining of any neck pain," I said, remembering all his protests about having the collar on. If I had listened. . . .

"I know. That's not unusual. We just did this X ray as part of our routine to make sure his neck was all right before we removed the collar."

"Holy shit." I called Dave and Tim over and together we stared at the X ray. "Great job, guys," I said. "I used to think that EMTs couldn't actually kill anyone, just fail to save them. In this case one wrong move. . . ."

I returned to my car and, by the time I arrived back at my house, Joan was waiting for me. As I told her about the call, I sank into a chair. "I never really appreciated the seriousness of something like this."

Later that evening, we drove back to the hospital and found Dr. Morrison, still on duty. "I'm glad you stopped back," he said. "I wanted to ask you for a few more details about the accident." He asked about the condition of both cars, and I told him as much as I knew. Then he said, "I understand he had no lap belt."

"Just that shoulder harness," I said. "Do you think that was what broke his neck?"

"Yeah. He was probably forced down under the dash and the shoulder harness caught his chin and snapped his head back. You saw the deep laceration under his jaw?"

"Yeah, I did. Can Joan see that X ray?"

"Sure," Dr. Morrison said, and he led us to the display where Nomad's X rays were still posted. While Joan stared at the picture, Dr. Morrison pointed to the X ray of Nomad's leg. "And here's the femur. Look at the amount of displacement." I looked and easily saw that Nomad's left thigh bone had been broken in half and the ends overlapped by several inches. "He's also got a left pneumothorax from a cracked rib. He's one sick guy, but he'll be okay."

"Will he have to wear one of those halo things to support his neck?" Joan asked.

"No. He'll be here for quite a while with his neck protected and then he'll be in a hard collar for about three months. But he will eventually be fine."

"That's good," I said.

"And listen, Ed. Convey my congratulations to your crew. You guys did a great job on this one." When I stared at him, he added quickly, "As you always do, of course."

A few weeks later there was a letter posted on the bulletin board.

To an EMT named Ed and the rest of the ambulance crew who came to my husband's aid after his accident:

Thank you all so very much. Nomad tells me that he wasn't so nice to all of you. I can tell you that he was always complaining about things, even before the accident. But he's coming home from the hospital soon and I look forward to listening to his complaints from his own room.

The doctor tells me that if you people hadn't been so careful he might have died. That really scares us both.

Thank you so much!

The note was signed "Evelyn Kobelev."

Sometimes the most important things that EMTs do have nothing to do with what is learned in classrooms. I don't think of myself as being particularly good with children. It has been more than twenty years since my own daughters were small, and I don't really remember how to talk to little ones. When Joan and I are on a pediatric call together, I usually back off and let her handle it. Joan is a former schoolteacher and seems to be able to establish an instant rapport with children. But sometimes Joan is not around.

It was a Saturday afternoon and I was out in the garden, pulling weeds. The salvias, nicotianas, and petunias I had planted in the spring to attract ruby-throated hummingbirds now seemed to be in mortal danger from the weeds that were spreading wildly in the midsummer heat. As my fire department pager began to beep, I threw down the handful of oxalis and crabgrass that I had pulled out of the flower bed and listened.

"GVK–861 to the rescue squad. A full crew is needed to respond to the Prescott Gymnastics Center for a child with head and neck injuries. Will a full crew please call in. GVK–861, clear."

I sprinted into the house, grabbed the phone, and pushed the Prescott Fire speed-dial button.

"Prescott Fire Department, Rizzo speaking."

"Hi, Andy. It's Ed Herman. I'll respond to the firehouse as the EMT."

"Okay, Ed. Max Taylor just called in as the driver, and Les Kravitski will meet you at the scene."

It was not surprising that a crew had called in so quickly. It was a Saturday and the call was for a child with a possibly serious injury. I wiped my hands and ran to the car. Switching on the blue courtesy light, I carefully backed out of my driveway and headed for the fire station. Max lived right around the corner from my house, and a couple of near collisions had taught both of us to be extra careful at the bottom of my driveway when responding to rescue calls.

Paramedic Hugh Washington had already been on the scene for about five minutes by the time we rolled the rig to a stop in front of the Prescott Gymnastics Center. He met me at the entrance as I stepped out of the ambulance. Behind him stood a man in his early thirties, holding a little girl, whose face was pressed against his shoulder.

"Hi, Hugh," I said. "What have you got?"

"The girl was doing a somersault off a seven-foot-high platform and didn't tuck her head enough when she landed on the mat. She landed on her face."

"What kind of injuries?"

"Well, her nose was bleeding and it's a bit swollen but there's no deformity. Her father says that he thinks she may have injured her neck." Hugh nodded toward the man holding the child. Noticing the implied question on my face Hugh added, "The little girl won't let anyone but her father near her. There's no way she will allow any kind of immobilization. I'm afraid that if you try to immobilize her, you'll just make any neck or back injury worse. You'll have to transport her with her father holding her."

"Is there any indication of a head injury?" I asked.

"Not that I could see, but she wouldn't let me examine her."

"How about point tenderness in the neck or back?"

"She wouldn't let me palpate."

"Did you get any vitals?"

"Look, Ed, the kid started to scream and thrash whenever I tried to touch her. Just get her over to the hospital. Okay?" he said, starting to get annoyed with my questions.

I was a bit surprised at Hugh's cavalier attitude but I knew from a few other calls we had been on together that he was not very good with children. "Okay, Hugh," I said. "You're absolutely right. I won't fight with her. If I have to, I'll transport her in her father's arms. I just wanted as much information as possible."

While I spoke with Hugh, Les Kravitski arrived, led the man holding the child into the ambulance, and got him comfortably seated on the stretcher. As I climbed into the rig, Les asked, "Do you want me to come along, Ed? I have a really full day, but I'll come if you need me."

"Thanks, Les, but I think the fewer the people, the less upset the child will be. I shouldn't have any trouble handling it alone."

"Great." As Les closed the door of the ambulance, I turned toward the little girl whose face was still pressed against her father's shoulder. I didn't want to transport her in that position without even knowing her state of consciousness, so I began speaking to her. "Hi, my name is Ed," I said gently, positioning myself so that she would be able to see me with as little head movement as possible. She turned her head slightly and peered at me. I wasn't happy about her turning her head, but in the position that she was in, the ambulance ride could be at least as dangerous as the slight head movement. "Can you tell me your name?" I asked.

"It's Caroline," the man said.

"I'd like to have your daughter answer herself," I explained to the man.

"Oh, sure," he replied.

"Hi, Caroline," I continued. "I'm pleased to meet you. Can you tell me how old you are?"

The little girl peered at me suspiciously. "I'm gonna be five," she said in a surprisingly strong voice.

"Almost five? Wow. That's pretty old. Does that mean you'll be starting kindergarten this fall?"

"Yes," she answered.

I turned to the girl's father. "Did you pick her up off of the floor after she fell?"

"No. She ran over to me, screaming. I grabbed her while the counselor called 911."

Good news, I thought. She had been moving all four limbs after the accident. "I understand you hurt yourself while doing gymnastics," I said. "Can you tell me what you like to do in gymnastics?"

Within a few minutes I had established a dialogue with Caroline, and she seemed to be losing her fear of me. It was apparent that her level of consciousness was normal and there did not seem to be any need to rush to the hospital.

Max, sitting in the driver's seat, looked over his shoulder at me. "You ready to go, Ed?"

"No. Give me a few minutes," I replied.

I reached into the box of latex gloves, pulled one out,

and showed it to the little girl. "Do you know what this is?" I asked.

"It's a glove," she replied.

"Would you like to see me turn this glove into a balloon?"

"Yes," she replied, sure that I was teasing her but curious nevertheless.

I held the opening of the glove against my mouth and blew into it. Caroline's eyes widened as she watched the glove inflate. Then her face broke into a smile.

"Would you like to have this balloon?" I asked, tying off the hand opening.

"Yes," she replied, now beaming.

I handed Caroline the inflated glove with the thumb pointed toward her and the other fingers forming a crest along the top. "You know, this sort of looks like a rooster to me," I said. "It has a beak and a comb on its head, but we'll have to give it eyes and a mouth when we get to the hospital. Okay?"

"Okay," she agreed.

"Caroline, can you tell me where you're hurt?" I asked.

Having been reminded of her injury, Caroline began to whimper. "My nose hurts."

"Can you show me where?"

Caroline pointed to the tip of her nose. I could see that it was slightly swollen, but there was just a tiny bit of dried blood on her upper lip and neither deformation nor discoloration. I doubted that it was broken. Since there were only a few drops of blood on the girl's clothes, it was obvious that the bleeding had been minor.

"Caroline, does your neck or back hurt?" I asked.

"No," she replied as if I had asked a foolish question. "Just my nose."

"Do you hurt anywhere else?"

The little girl looked at me as if I were teasing her and giggled. "No. I told you. Just my nose."

"Well, that's great," I said. "I'm glad you're not hurt anywhere else. May I examine your neck and back?" The question was crucial. If she would allow me to touch her, I would be able to get the information that I needed before starting the bumpy ride to the hospital. I didn't know what I would do, however, if I found evidence of a neck or back injury. Spinal immobilization involves having your head and body tied down to a board. It is uncomfortable and produces anxiety even in adults. Despite the trust that I was beginning to achieve with Caroline, I doubted that she would ever submit to a spinal immobilization without a struggle. And such a struggle could do more damage than transporting her without immobilization. But I would try if necessary.

"Caroline, I want you to tell me if it hurts anywhere when I touch you," I said, gently palpating her neck and back.

"Okay," she replied.

There was no tenderness and no deformity anywhere along her spinal column, and within a short time I was able to determine that the little girl had full movement and sensation in her hands and feet. An examination of her pupils revealed a normal reaction to light. There was no evidence of any spinal injury, and there would be no reason not to transport her in her father's arms. Caroline was now fully cooperative and allowed me to do a complete body survey, obtain a full set of vitals, and use my stethoscope to listen to her lung sounds. Within a few minutes we were able to begin our trip to Fairfax General Hospital.

While waiting for the doctor to examine Caroline at the hospital, I took a swab, dipped it in Betadine solution, and painted brown eyes and a smiling mouth on the glove balloon. "That's a funny-looking rooster," Caroline commented about my artwork.

Max came in and handed her a paper. "You were so brave that this is an application for you to become a firefighter," he explained.

"I'm too little to be a firefighter." Caroline giggled.

"Well, you can be a junior firefighter," Max said. "We need more women in our fire department."

Having completed our paperwork and put clean linen on the stretcher, we walked toward the big automatic ER doors. As we passed the room in which Dr. Margolis was examining Caroline, we heard her say to her father, "Daddy, I want to be a firefighter when I grow up." Except for her bruised nose, Caroline was found to be uninjured and was released to go home with her father.

We're called "volunteers," but that doesn't mean that we volunteer for each emergency medical call that we respond to. As members of the Fairfax Volunteer Ambulance Corps, we are required to ride at least four six-hour duty shifts every month. While on duty we take whatever call comes in, be it an intoxicated person who has fallen and is vomiting, a drug overdose, a teenager who broke his hand in a fight, a terminal cancer patient needing transport, or a person who is simply using the ambulance as a taxi service to the hospital. And we treat them all in a calm and "professional" manner, with respect and courtesy if not always with sympathy. But sometimes it can be very difficult.

Joan and I had often seen Cindy Black around town. Cindy was in her fifties, her long black hair streaked with gray. She had obviously been a strikingly attractive woman when she was younger, but her face was now frozen into an expression of anger. She carried a small folding chair around under her arm and usually would open it and sit in front of one of the large stores and sell pencils or other trinkets to people entering and leaving. She was aggressive and would glare at shoppers and virtually demand that they buy something from her. She was also aggressively vocal about her racial beliefs. Among others, she hated Jews, Blacks, Hispanics, Poles, and homosexuals, although not necessarily in that order. Joan and I referred to her, between ourselves, as the Nazi and tried to avoid her as much as possible. But it wasn't always possible.

Joan and I were on the midnight to 6 A.M. duty shift, and it was 3:30 in the morning when the telephone rang. Maybe it's a wrong number, I thought as I picked up the phone. "Hello," I said.

"Hi, Ed, it's Will McAndrews at the police department. We have an unknown medical at the Hillcrest Apartments, room 354A. Pete Williamson is at the corps and he's responding with the rig."

"Okay, Will. Joan and I will respond to the scene."

We threw on our FVAC uniforms, ran to the car, and drove to the Hillcrest Apartments, about a mile away.

The ambulance was just ahead of us as we pulled into the apartment complex driveway and stopped in front of the main entrance. As we got out of the car, I could see

Cindy, sitting on her chair at the curb with a small suit-case on the pavement next to her.

"Oh, shit," I whispered to Joan.

"It's all right," Joan replied. "I'll be crew chief. Let's see whether Pete will get in back and you can drive."

"Thanks," I said as we climbed out of the car.

"Hi," Joan said. "I'm Joan and this is Ed and that's Pete. You're Cindy Black, right?"

"Yeah."

"What seems to be the matter, Cindy?" she asked. Joan could be pleasant to a serial killer, I thought. Out of the corner of my eye I saw that Pete was retrieving the stretcher from the back of the ambulance.

"It's my arm. I got this rash," Cindy replied, holding out her arm for Joan to inspect.

"How long have you had a rash?" Joan asked, looking at the arm in the light from the front of the apartment complex's door.

"A couple of months." A couple of months, I thought. That's just wonderful. It's almost 4:00 A.M.

"Are you having any other problems?"

"Nah, just the rash. It itches and I can't sleep."

"Well, why did you call us tonight?" Joan asked.

"I ran out of my prescription ointment."

"Why didn't you get some yesterday, before you ran out?"

"Those Jew pharmacists are crooks. You know what they charge for a little tube of ointment? Five and a half bucks. At the hospital I get it for free."

"Yeah, I see your point," I began sarcastically, but Joan cut me off.

"Why don't you go and get ready to drive, Ed?" she said. "Pete and I will take care of Cindy."

I began to protest but quickly realized that we would all be better off with me away from our patient. Silently I waited behind the wheel and waited until Joan and Pete had gotten Cindy comfortable on the stretcher. "Don't lose my chair!" I heard Cindy snap. I watched in the side mirror as Pete folded Cindy's chair and stowed it in the rig.

"Okay, Ed," Joan finally said. "We're ready to go."

"Fairfax General?" I asked.

"No. She wants to go down to St. Luke's Trauma Center. Her doctor's there."

That figures, I thought. Fairfax General was less than ten minutes away. St. Luke's was about thirty minutes away from this part of town.

"Lights and siren?" I asked sarcastically.

"No, Ed. No lights and no siren. Just take it code 2, nice and easy," Joan replied. I knew that she knew what I was feeling and I hoped she would excuse my fury.

While en route to the hospital, I could hear snatches of conversation from the back of the ambulance.

"Are you people Jewish?" Cindy asked.

"Pete here isn't but Ed and I are."

"Oh," Cindy said. "I get along well with Jews. You people are so smart. And you always stick together. The last time the ambulance took me to the hospital, the EMT who took care of me was Italian. I can't stand those Italians. They're so damn pushy. He tried to tell me I didn't need an ambulance. Some nerve, huh?"

It was after 5:00 A.M. and beginning to get light when Joan and I finally staggered back to bed after dealing with Cindy's rash. I like to think that, had I been crew chief, I would have been as polite, respectful, and professional as Joan was throughout that ambulance call, but I'm not at all sure that I would have had as much self-control.

Like all towns, Fairfax has its characters, and Cindy isn't the only one.

Louis the Gangster was the terror of all Fairfax town service providers. Louis was eighty-two years old, short, stocky, and wheelchair bound. He had a mechanized wheelchair, which he had somehow "souped up" so that it was able to travel at speeds that no wheelchair was ever meant to go. In his youth, Louis had been a mechanic and a dock worker. He claimed that, later in his life, he had been an enforcer for "the mob," and since he seemed particularly proud of that period, he made sure that everyone who came into contact with him knew about it. It was not unusual for Louis to threaten us when we were on one of our frequent medical calls to his apartment in Hillcrest. "You sons of bitches drop me, you're gonna get busted heads. I still got connections with the mob."

The only time that Louis acted the least bit friendly was when he was asked about his life in the mob. Then he would have endless stories to tell, mostly of a violent nature. All of us at FVAC knew that the best way to get him to cooperate with us was simply to say "Hey, Louis, tell my partner about that time on the dock when that guy came at you with the ice pick." Louis would launch into a story, liberally sprinkled with four-letter words, and would act like a pussy cat all the way to the hospital.

For the Fairfax Police, however, it wasn't that easy. Louis hated cops. One of his favorite pastimes was careening his wheelchair down the center of Route 10.

I would frequently hear the police dispatcher on my scanner: "325 to 703."

"703 on."

"Respond over to Route 10 in the vicinity of the entrance to Harry S. Truman State Park. We have a report of Louis the . . . of an elderly gentleman driving a wheelchair down the middle of the road."

"10–4," a weary voice would answer. "703 is responding code 3."

The police would respond as quickly as possible whenever they received a complaint about Louis from an incredulous citizen, hoping to stop him before he either caused an accident or was himself injured. Over the years, both had happened a number of times. But stopping him wasn't easy, since Louis would ignore the police car sirens and their demands that he pull over. He would take evasive maneuvers and try to outrun them. When they finally managed to stop him, Louis would curse and swing at them as they approached his wheelchair. "No fuckin' cop is gonna take me alive," he would yell. The police would have to arrest him, wheelchair and all. Inevitably, however, whether taken to the hospital or the town lockup, Louis would be out and careening around town in his wheelchair within a few days, endangering his own life and those of his fellow citizens.

Over the years, since he lived alone, Louis became a "regular," and I had responded to his apartment several times. A few times he'd fallen out of his wheelchair and he just needed help to get back in. I responded one morning when he had been on the floor for almost a full day. On that occasion, in addition to his deteriorated condition due to his long stay on the floor, he seemed to have some weakness on his right side. I remember wondering at that time whether he'd be able to operate the controls of his wheelchair if that arm was, indeed, weakened by a stroke. But weakened or not, he cursed all the way to the hospital, yelling at us because we hadn't been able to get his powered wheelchair in the ambulance. "How the hell am I going to be able to get around? You could have fit my chair in here. Look at all this room."

I discovered later that Louis had indeed had a stroke and had been transferred to a nursing home. Louis the Gangster died there about a month ago. I sort of miss him.

As an EMT I often get to see the less attractive aspects of humanity. Drunken drivers, spouse and child abusers, and people who habitually misuse the EMS system sometimes cause me to have a rather jaundiced eye toward my fellow citizens. But then, just when I'm really down on people, I have an EMS experience that makes it impossible for me to remain a confirmed misanthrope.

It had been one of those days that I think of as a "reverse Midas" day—a day when everything I touched seemed to turn to mud, or worse. It was midsummer, hot and humid. I had just finished cleaning up after dropping a bottle filled with iced tea. The bottle had shattered, leaving puddles of tea and shards of glass all over my kitchen floor. I had finally settled myself on my deck and was trying to read and understand a highly technical article about a new method to genetically engineer plants. I was late completing the August issue of the plant biotechnology newsletter that I write and publish and was feeling under pressure to finish, which made concentrating even more difficult.

I found myself reading the same sentence over and over again. Suddenly my pager began to beep. "GVK–861 to the rescue squad. A full crew is needed for a PIAA at the intersection of Judy and Maple."

It was a personal injury automobile accident. I decided to ignore the pager. Just because I work at home doesn't mean I have to take every call that comes in, I thought. If I break my concentration, it will take me an hour to get back to where I am. Besides, other EMTs are usually quick to respond to automobile accidents. I tried to continue reading.

The pager sounded again. "GVK–861 to the rescue squad. An EMT and an attendant are still needed for a PIAA at the intersection of Judy and Maple. Will an EMT and an attendant please call in."

It is always difficult to cover weekday calls during the hours when our volunteers are at work. During August it is even more difficult because a lot of rescue squad members are away on vacation. If Prescott can't raise a crew the dispatcher will have to call FVAC for mutual aid, I thought, and they're having as much trouble covering day calls as we are.

The pager beeped again. "GVK–861 to the rescue squad. This is your third and final page. An EMT and an attendant are still needed for a PIAA at the intersection of Judy and Maple. Will an EMT and an attendant please call in."

Oh, well, I thought, I'm not having much luck concentrating anyway. So the issue will be another day late. I threw my papers down and headed for the telephone.

Les Kravitski was behind the wheel of the rig, waiting for me as I pulled into the firehouse parking lot. I popped open my trunk, grabbed my stethoscope, turnout coat, and helmet, and jumped into the ambulance. Even though the temperature was in the nineties, our safety rules require that I wear my turnout coat and helmet if I have to get into a wrecked car to help a patient.

"It's just the two of us," Les said as, siren wailing, we pulled out of the ambulance bay. "Nobody called in as an attendant and there are two victims. The medic at the scene reports minor injuries and says that we can take both patients in one rig."

"Oh, great," I said. "That's just what I needed today. Just me alone with two patients."

I wouldn't be alone at the scene. Les was a good EMT and there would be a medic there as well as a number of firefighters. Although the firefighters weren't EMTs, they were great at extricating accident victims and assisting with spinal immobilizations. But if it was a BLS call—a situation in which the paramedics weren't needed—I would end up alone in the back of the ambulance, responsible for two patients. Therefore, my name would be at the bottom of the prehospital care report as the person "in charge" even though there was no way that I could simultaneously supervise the evaluation, extrication, immobilization, and treatment of two victims at the same time. If there were ever a lawsuit and the PCR was introduced as evidence, I would be the one who would have to explain and justify everything that had been done.

I just hoped that the two patients would not be the drivers of two cars that had collided with each other. That could be an explosive situation. In the past, on more than one occasion, I had had to deal with two drivers who screamed and cursed at each other all the way to the hospital from adjacent stretchers while lying on their backs, strapped to longboards.

We were about a half mile from the scene when the ambulance's engine suddenly stopped. "Damn," Les muttered. "It's dead."

The ambulance rolled to a stop. Les cranked the starter over and over again until, finally, it restarted. Pulling out onto the road, Les grabbed the radio microphone. "21–02 to GVK–861," he called.

"Go ahead, Rescue 2," the dispatcher replied.

"Respond with another rig to the scene. This rig just dropped dead for no reason. I got it started again but it will have to go out of service until we figure out what's wrong."

"10–4, Rescue 2. We'll get someone to drive 21–03 to the scene."

"And put FVAC on standby at their headquarters since we'll have no rigs available," Les added.

"Will do," the dispatcher replied.

We were only a few hundred feet from the accident scene and could see the lights of the emergency vehicles when the ambulance died again. This time Les could not restart it.

"Let's just leave the rig here. It's off the road and we can walk from here. Why don't you grab a longboard and I'll get a KED and spider straps," I said.

We quickly gathered the equipment and jogged over to the middle of the intersection where two cars rested with their front ends intimately intertwined. Paramedic Amy Chen was putting a cervical collar around the neck of an elderly man in the driver's seat of one car.

"Hi, Amy," I said. "What have you got?"

Amy turned toward me. "Hi, Ed. This is an eighty-three-year-old male complaining of pain to the left ribs. He apparently made a left turn directly into the path of the other car. His chest is intact, lung sounds are clear, and vitals are within normal limits."

"Did you check out the driver of the other car?" I asked.

"Yeah. The driver is a twenty-eight-year-old female. She's got a seat-belt abrasion to her chest and is complaining of some abdominal pain and pain in her knee. Her lung sounds and vitals are good also and there's no abdominal rigidity or point tenderness. They can both go BLS." Basic life support. No need for a paramedic.

"Any signs or symptoms of spinal injury?" I asked, nodding toward the cervical collar that Amy had just applied.

"No. There's no neurological deficit or any neck or back problems."

"Great, Amy, but I'm the only EMT here and we need to immobilize both patients. Can you stay with this one and supervise his extrication while I take care of the other?"

"Sure, Ed. As long as we don't get another call."

Within a short time we had extricated both accident victims, immobilized them on longboards, and loaded them into the ambulance. Alone with the two drivers in the back of 21–03, I took a moment to gather information and take vitals. The driver who had brought –03 to the scene would stay with the still-dead –02 until the tow truck arrived. Les was filling him in on Rescue 2's "symptoms" and then would drive us to the hospital.

I started to write down the patients' names and addresses. The elderly man, who had been calm and silent as I helped him from the vehicle, answered in a soft voice; he was visibly shaken. It had been clear to everyone that the accident had been his fault. The woman had been upset despite attempts by a state police officer, firefighters, and myself to reassure her. She was still crying as we began to roll toward Fairfax General Hospital.

"Elizabeth," I said softly to her once I finished writing, "try to calm down."

Suddenly the man said softly, "I'm so sorry, Elizabeth."

Elizabeth stopped crying and the inside of the ambulance was silent for a few seconds. Then the young woman reached across the narrow space between the two stretchers and took his hand. "That's all right," she said. "It was just an accident. Accidents happen to everyone."

"But—" He began to sob softly.

"It's all right," Elizabeth said. "I'm going to be just fine and so are you."

Despite the fact that they were both totally immobilized, flat on their backs on hard wooden boards, the elderly man and the young woman held hands all the way to the hospital, where they were both treated and released.

By the time I got back to my house, an afternoon thunderstorm had cooled the air. Before resuming my work, I spent a few minutes relaxing and replaying the rescue call in my mind. Maybe people aren't so bad, I thought. I found that I was now able to concentrate on my work and got the August issue of my newsletter finished without further delay.

Chapter 8

Since the publication of our first book, *Rescue Alert,* five years ago, we have received a lot of letters from people involved in EMS. Many contained stories. With their permission, here are some of those tales, told as the writers told them to us with just names and locations changed.

I'm a paramedic and my EMT cohort and I had been called to the scene of a possible heart attack. We arrived along with Officer Forenz in his police cruiser. We began to treat the patient, a sixty-two-year-old woman with chest pains, with high-flow oxygen and I set up to start a line. It took a while to get the IV established. We were almost ready to transport so I put in a call to the hospital to report and get orders.

Dimly in the background I heard the officer get a call on his radio. He said something to my partner and dashed out the door. "Rob," my partner said to me. "Tell the doc that transport will be delayed."

"Why?" I asked.

"I'll explain later. Just tell him we'll be delayed another six or seven minutes."

I relayed the message to the doc at the hospital, and he decided to give our patient nitro. I hung up and got a nitro from the drug box. "Place this under your tongue," I told the patient. "Don't chew it or swallow it. Just let it dissolve." As she placed the tiny pill beneath her tongue, I turned to Mike. "What's this about delayed transport?"

"The rig's gone."

"What?"

"The call the cop got was from someone a few blocks away, asking why there was an ambulance in her driveway with the lights flashing. I've called for a second rig in case the first is damaged. I also thought they might want evidence or something."

The second ambulance arrived and we quickly transported our patient. We met Officer Forenz at the hospital. "This guy's drunk and leaves the party he's at to take a walk. He walks, waters several lawns along the way, then forgets where the party was. So he takes the ambulance to look around. Needless to say, he finds the house, puts the rig in the neighbor's driveway, jumps into his pickup, and heads home."

"You're kidding," Mike and I said in unison.

"Nope," Officer Forenz said. "He's out of our jurisdiction now, so we've got local authorities en route to pick him up."

"How'd you find all this out?"

"Actually I visited the location where the party was and talked to the two women who answered the door. They told me they knew nothing about nothing."

"So how'd you get the story?"

"I simply told them that if your patient died they could be charged with murder. Real quick they knew everything."

* * *

This from an EMT in New Mexico. He was new to EMS when this incident happened.

I was doing an internship as a firefighter with a rural fire department in northwest Oregon. We were dispatched to a logging road for a report of an all-terrain-vehicle accident. As we parked the ambulance at the end of the road, we were met by a couple of men with five horses. The patient had rolled his ATV in an area that was almost inaccessible and, we were told, the best way to get there was on horseback. Since we lived in a rural area, most of us had at least some time on horseback, so we mounted up and headed out. Jim, the only medic on duty, was carrying the jump kit and I had the oxygen and airway supplies. The trauma gear and immobilization equipment were split among the other three.

We left the road and headed up a steep hill through the trees, led by one of the patient's friends. Jim, looking very much the part of a cowboy, gave his horse a good kick to catch up with us. To the surprise of everyone, including the medic, Jim's horse decided he'd had enough of the hard work, so he turned around and headed back down the hill at a full gallop. Fortunately, Jim had the presence of mind to drop the jump kit before he disappeared down the hill. We retrieved the kit and proceeded up to the patient, packaged him on a longboard, made a travois—an Indian-style stretcher—and towed him back to the ambulance. Jim was nowhere to be found.

After transporting the patient to the hospital, we returned to the station to find Jim's horse tied up in back.

We all went upstairs to find Jim, in the recliner, covered with scrapes and scratches, mumbling, "Damn, fucking horses. Never again. Damn, fucking horses."

At the annual Department Awards Ceremony Jim received the first, and to my knowledge the only, Roy Rogers Award for Bravery.

This story came to us from an eighteen-year-old from New Jersey. She begins her letter saying that she's been an EMT and a firefighter for about two years.

One incident still haunts me. It was the summer of 1996. My boyfriend and I were returning from a relaxing weekend at the shore. We both were extremely tired and the traffic was a mess. I closed my eyes and began to dream of the sands moving between my toes. My dream started to fade when I heard my boyfriend calling my name. As I opened my eyes my boyfriend's face was blank. He just stared out the front windshield and said, "Oh my God."

As I followed his eyes I saw a man lying in the narrow road. When I looked across the roadway I saw two people climbing out of a truck that had hit a tree. I remember unfastening my safety belt and yelling at my boyfriend to get my crash kit.

I jumped out of the car and began to run toward the accident. I knew some of the things to do, but, you see, I was just going to start my EMT class the following Monday.

As I approached I saw a male about thirty-five years old. I bent over and found that he was unconscious and not breathing. He appeared to be missing part of his skull and brain. The rest of his body was twisted: His right foot was pointing inward, his knee near his thigh. It was hard to cope.

I had two choices. I could start CPR and pray to God that he might have a chance or get started on the others. Well, I don't need to say what my choice was. I just left him lying in the roadway and did what I could for the people from the truck who were injured.

About a month after the accident I drove by the same spot to find a sign that read "In loving memory of Daddy, the best man in my life." Reading that nearly killed me. Up until recently I felt so guilty and unsure about my decision. You see, I felt so helpless. It has taken me a long time to accept the fact that there was really nothing I could have done for the man. Now I look at all the good that I've done since then, from the most minor situations to some serious ones. I'm still new and I grow up every day.

We received this wonderful tale from a female EMT in Alabama.

Our town is small and usually pretty quiet. One Sunday afternoon we were called out for a "kid stuck in a creek." We respond from our homes, so the driver and I met at the ambulance and were given directions.

The call was way out in the country and it took almost ten minutes to find the dirt road the dispatcher had described to us. As we bounced along we were talking, trying to figure out what we were needed for. We thought maybe a four-wheeler or something like that rolled over on a kid, trapping him underneath it.

We got to a bridge with about four people standing there looking over the side. The scene was safe so we got out, looked over the side and, sure enough, there was a fifteen-year-old kid in the water below. He waved. It turns out that he had been fishing and walked down to the edge of the water. Then his footing gave way and he sunk up to his waist in clay, sand, and water. He didn't need medical help, he was just stuck. Really stuck! The muck was like quicksand, but the kid wasn't sinking. He just couldn't get out. Trying to keep straight faces, my partner and I worked our way to him. Actually we had to use three backboards placed side by side so we would not get stuck too.

We tried pulling on the kid's legs but that didn't work. Neither did trying to dig his feet out. As we dug, the goo just refilled the hole as fast as we shoveled. My partner had a good idea. We put a KED on the boy, whose name was Jake, tied ropes from the jacket to the bridge, and pulled. No luck.

A little snake came swimming by and everyone, except the kid, scattered. After it swam away, we got back to work.

At that point we had about eight people working with us and a dozen or so on the bank and bridge offering suggestions. The kid was fine, by the way, making jokes and laughing with us, but there seemed to be no way of getting him out.

It had been almost two hours when someone came up with the idea of using a fire truck and a water hose for counterpressure. I wasn't exactly sure what that meant, but I was willing to go along with any "bright idea."

Someone went and called the FD and we waited until a truck arrived. Several firefighters piled out of the engine, looked over the edge of the bridge, and laughed. Finally they dropped a one-inch hose to us and we ran it down beside the kid's legs. The driver turned the pressure on low and I pulled. Bingo. The water pressure broke the suction and one leg was free. We propped him up on our long backboard and moved the hose. Shortly thereafter the second leg was free. We got his shoes and socks off to check pulses and everything was fine. He walked up the embankment, his mom signed my refusal paper, and we gathered up equipment to head back to the station.

We were all so dirty, we had to use the hose on both the ambulance and each other.

The same woman also sent us this story.

One Saturday night about midnight my husband and I were called out for a guy who was bleeding from the head. We were told to respond to the police station. Right then I should have prepared myself for the worst. Any pickups from the police station are usually trouble.

We got up, dressed, and drove to headquarters. We picked up the ambulance and, when we arrived at the police station, there was a guy sitting outside with a small open wound on his forehead. There was no active bleeding but the guy, who seemed to be in his early thirties, was very, very drunk. I asked him whether he was our patient and he said, "Yes," so I began my workup.

Moments later my husband and the police chief came out of the building and informed me that this guy, who told me his name was Slick and refused to give me any more information, was not the patient that we had been called for. He did need to go to the hospital with us, however, so someone could check out his head injury. The chief explained that our real patient was at a nearby residence. I bandaged this guy's small head laceration while he kept fussing and yelling at me. I was a bit nervous about this drunk but, despite my request, no police officer was able to ride with us. Since he wasn't badly injured and I thought I'd need the stretcher for our real patient, I put him on the jump seat and buckled him in. Tight.

A third EMT arrived and I felt a bit more secure so, with him, the drunk, and me in the back, we drove to the designated house. Sure enough, our second patient, a man named Gary who was about the same age as the first, was also drunk, probably more so than Slick. We got him onto the stretcher and I noted a laceration to his forehead as well. Must have been a blue light special that night on head lacerations.

We lifted the stretcher into the rig and, as I began to bandage the second patient, the two men started yelling at each other. As they hollered, we began to understand. The reason they both had holes in their foreheads was that each had tried to beat the tar out of the other earlier in the evening.

We were still about fifteen minutes from the hospital when Slick opened his seat belt, dove over my partner, and attacked Gary. Boy, the fight was on! Fists, elbows, knees. My husband pulled the ambulance over and, since we had crossed into another jurisdiction, called for police backup from them. We didn't want to try to separate Slick and Gary in the small back of the ambulance so we just stepped back and let things progress. When the cops arrived, they got the guys apart and back into their proper places. It took a few more gauze pads and a bit more tape to cover the new scrapes and contusions on each of them.

The police followed as far as they could, but we finally left their territory too.

Having heard what was going on, a third local police force called us and asked whether we still needed help. "Yes!" we answered. When we pulled into the emergency room there were four police officers lined up across the dock waiting for us.

This was one night we didn't have to unload our patients. They got a police escort right into the emergency room.

An EMT, firefighter, and specialist in extrication who lives and rides in Iowa sent this story.

It was early in the spring and the weather outside was rather cold. It had been raining for the last few days, leaving a depressing fog over the town. I sat on the side of a bathtub in an apartment the company I worked for owned, cussing the soldering job I had just finished. The damn tub was still leaking and I wasn't having any luck stopping it. Our department pagers sounded for an ambulance call somewhere in the city but I paid very little attention to it. I had to finish the job since the new tenants were moving in a few hours later. They covered the call quickly and, relieved, I returned to swearing at the still-leaking tub. A few minutes later the pagers sounded again and I paid a little more attention. Knowing that most of the available day crew had taken the earlier run, I set down my torch and listened to the dispatcher announce there was an MVA, a motor vehicle accident, on the interstate and that an ambulance was involved.

Oh, shit, I thought. Our rig had just left for the hospital

with the patient from the earlier run and had no doubt taken the interstate to get to the hospital fifteen minutes away. I ran from the apartment while cleaning my hands with waterless soap I carry for such occurrences. I jumped into my car and tossed the blue light onto the dash. Being about five minutes from the station, I had plenty of time to think. We had just put the new ambulance into service and this was one of its first calls. At that moment all I could think was, Boy, is the chief going to be pissed if our new rig is scratched!

As I pulled into the fire station parking lot, the second due ambulance passed me on the way to the MVA. I ran into the station and asked one of the fire lieutenants whether indeed it was our rig in the accident. I was relieved to hear that it wasn't ours, but rather a rig from a private paramedic service in the next town. That relief was cut short by the information that people were trapped in the vehicle and that CPR was in progress on at least one patient. Having missed the ambulance, I ran to my fire gear hanging on the rack and pulled on my boots and pants. A few more people had arrived by this time and we jumped into the rescue truck, which carries all the extrication equipment, and headed for the scene. While pulling on my heavy fire coat I announced over the radio that we were en route.

The next radio traffic I heard brought more bad news. Neither of the air ambulances in the area were flying due to the lousy weather. Bad things seemed to get worse at every opportunity. Traffic was terrible and even with air horn and siren blasting, it seemed to take an eternity to get to the location of the accident.

As we crested a hill the scene that greeted me is one I will never forget. There in the middle lane was an ambulance in shattered ruins. It was resting on the driver's side looking like some sort of wounded animal. Our second due ambulance was on the scene and, as we drove around large piles of debris, I saw that the crew was working on a patient at the side of the road. I jumped out of the rescue truck, pulled on my helmet, and was immediately grabbed by one of the local tow truck drivers who asked me for a wrench to shut off the gas on the overturned ambulance. I gave him the tool box from the rescue and went to see who else was in need of assistance.

I took a quick look at the patient that several people were working on at the side of the road and determined that she was probably DRT (dead right there), but they had to continue work anyway. She was an elderly lady, wearing a hospital gown, obviously the patient from the ambulance. We needed the assistance of paramedics but as we were only a BLS unit, we would have to do our best without the benefit of a person who could administer drugs.

I next went to the overturned ambulance and looked into the back to find the attendant lying in a pile of broken medical equipment. A state trooper and a city police officer were providing aid to her, and I climbed in to help. While I worked on the woman, I could hear the lieutenant I came with at the front of the ambulance checking on the trapped driver and using his portable radio to call for mutual aid from one of the suburbs.

In what seemed like no time another rig had arrived, and I helped package and load the female attendant into it. She was pretty shaken up and was trying to tell me something but because of all the noise and confusion and the non-rebreather mask she was wearing I couldn't make out what it was.

As the ambulance pulled away I heard approaching sirens. I looked up to see our new ambulance pull up on the scene. Having dropped their patient off at the hospital they returned as quickly as they could to help us out. In addition, two state troopers came screaming along the breakdown lane to help divert traffic from the area and more of our town's fire officers were arriving to provide help also.

Then there was the most unbelievable sight of all. What appeared to be every rig from the private service whose ambulance had crashed was coming, code 3, to the scene. Paramedics! And lots of them! I turned in time to see our second ambulance crew load the CPR patient into their ambulance and head for the hospital with two paramedics on board.

Just when I thought everything was under control, I was approached by a man in a highway construction uniform. He asked if I had anything to pry the door off the truck his buddy was in. I looked several hundred feet down the road to where the highway crew dump truck sat in a ditch. Shit, I hadn't even noticed it on the way in.

I grabbed a Halligan tool and a pair of hand-operated spreaders out of the rescue truck. Since my lieutenant was using the jaws to free the driver of the ambulance this would have to do. I ran as best I could in all my fire gear to the dump truck and was glad to see that the door was already open. We quickly placed the driver in a C-collar and pulled him from the truck onto a long backboard. I then assisted two EMTs from the private ambulance service in loading him into one of their rigs. When they were gone I returned to the wrecked ambulance.

By now several rescue workers were inside the wreckage disassembling cabinets and moving equipment in the back in an attempt to get to the driver. The lieutenant and I used all of the power extrication equipment we had on the exterior, cutting away what we could, but we weren't having much luck. We discussed using a power saw to cut the roof off the ambulance, but it would be a time-consuming process.

As we stood talking, others continued using the tools. The news media arrived and several overanxious photographers began to get in our way in their attempt to get footage of the wreck for the noon news. When I saw them I could barely contain my anger. How anyone can get in the way of a rescue operation like that is beyond me.

I turned to the biggest, tallest of the state troopers near us and asked him to get the news guys out of there. He smiled, nodded, and extended one huge arm, pointing first at the cameramen and then to the side of the road. It was amazing that he didn't even need to say a word. His size and demeanor said it all. Sheepishly, still snapping pictures, they moved away. Just then the crew in the rig hollered that they had the driver freed from the debris, and we ran back to aid in his packaging and loading.

After all the ambulances had left for the hospital, I watched the tow truck crew lift the wrecked ambulance upright. A citizen who had been helping with the dump truck driver walked up to me and asked if we had something he could use to clean the blood off his hands. I walked with him back to our rescue truck and gave him some cleaning solution. He told me that he was also a volunteer firefighter and that he had been on his way to a job site for his full-time job. He said he saw the dump truck pull out from the side of the road, directly into the path of the approaching ambulance. With the weather making the road slick and the ambulance traveling at interstate speed, there was no way the driver could have avoided the accident.

We collected our gear, checked that we had all our tools, and returned to the station. While I was there cleaning up, the medical director for the private ambulance service arrived to thank us for our hard work. He had the crushed remains of the defibrillator along with smashed drug boxes and jump kits from the rig with him. We all sat around a table filled with the crushed equipment. Everyone was silent, lost in thought over the accident and thinking how easily it could have been one of us. The medical director told us that the rig had been transporting a patient between hospitals and that the elderly woman had not been in very good condition to begin with. He also told us how, when he heard the call and realized that it was one of his units involved, he had dispatched all his available paramedic units to the scene and then manned the fly car himself.

A few minutes later the phone rang and my lieutenant took the call. It was one of our crews at the hospital. The woman on whom they had been doing CPR—the original ambulance patient—had been pronounced dead upon arrival. The dump truck driver had been taken to X ray, treated for minor injuries, and was in the process of being released. The female attendant in the ambulance was in serious condition and the driver was critical. Fortunately eventually both would recover fully. However, the female attendant decided to give up EMS. She went on to nursing school so she could work in a sane, nonmoving environment.

The bathtub probably still leaks.

* * *

And this was told to us by a friend who has nothing to do with EMS. It happened to a friend of hers.

Although he had studied English for several years at the Unversité de Paris and had visited England several times, this was Eduard Chevreau's first trip to the United States. Eduard regularly read English-language magazines and newspapers and prided himself on his knowledge of the language. He rarely, however, had an opportunity to practice his spoken English, as few of his friends or business associates spoke the language. This week, however, he was determined not to speak French at all.

He had arrived from Paris the previous day for a week-long vacation in the United States. He and his son Antoine, who was a graduate student at New York University, were going to spend the week at a cabin in Vermont. Eduard had not seen Antoine in almost a year, and he was looking forward to being with his son, doing nothing but fishing and sailing on Bluebird Lake.

Eduard and Antoine had stayed overnight with friends who lived in the town of Hastings-on-Hudson. In the morning they had driven north along the eastern shore of the Hudson River, past the magnificent old mansions overlooking the river, then though the village of Sleepy Hollow, where the headless horseman is said to have ridden. They had continued along the road cut into the side of Anthony's Nose, where the Hudson becomes a spectacular fjord as it winds through the Hudson Highlands, then past the cliffs of Breakneck Ridge.

It was late afternoon. With the sun roof open, they had

driven though Massachusetts and the southern part of Vermont and were approaching the rolling foothills of the Green Mountains. Eduard remembered reading about Ethan Allen and how his Green Mountain Boys had come down from the hills and had captured Fort Ticonderoga from the British before the American Revolution. Now the countryside was at peace and the forested hills were ablaze with the colors of early fall. Eduard calculated that they only had about half an hour before they would get to their cabin.

As Eduard maneuvered the rented car along the increasingly curvy highway, Antoine gazed at the brilliant reds and yellows of the sugar maples that covered the hills and lined the road. *"C'est magnifique. N'est-ce pas, Papa?"*

"Oui. Yes," his father replied. "Eet ees mahn-yee-fee-kuh."

Antoine laughed. "Okay, Papa," he said. "I'll speak English this week. But I'm so used to speaking French with you and Mama that it seems strange to be speaking English. Just remind me if I start speaking French again."

"I weel," Eduard assured his son. "By ze time I return to Paree, I want to be speaking English like a Yankee."

"Sure, Papa. You will have to learn French all over again."

Eduard and Antoine both chuckled as the car rounded a sharp curve.

Although Eduard had never seen one before, other than in pictures, he immediately recognized the heavy snout and the huge, flattened antlers of the beast that ran out of the woods, directly into the path of his car. Eduard slammed his foot on the brake and desperately pulled the steering wheel to the right, but it was too late. There was nothing he could do to avoid hitting the animal. He watched in horror as the beast was lifted by the front end of the car, slid along the hood, crashed through the windshield, and slid past him, over Antoine.

Eduard maneuvered the vehicle to a stop on the shoulder of the road, pulled up the emergency brake, and turned toward his son. The animal had slid all the way past Antoine and up through the sun roof where its shoulders were now lodged. The lower part of its body was on top of the younger man. Neither the animal nor Antoine was moving, and both were covered with shattered glass and blood. It was impossible to tell how much of the blood was from Antoine and how much was from the animal.

"Antoine, Antoine," Eduard yelled.

Antoine did not reply. Eduard reached over and shook his son. Both Antoine and the animal moved. "Antoine, *est-ce que ça va? Est-ce que tu es blessé?*"

Antoine remained silent.

Remembering that there was a cellular phone in the car, Eduard reached across the inert bodies of his son and the animal that lay on top of him and managed to get the glove compartment open just wide enough to reach the phone. Holding it, he hesitated for a few seconds, then remembered the U.S. emergency number. Eduard dialed 911.

Karen McFarly was approaching the end of her shift at the Highbridge Falls emergency dispatch center. It had been a relatively quiet day; the only real emergency had been a car fire. There had been, however, more than the usual number of annoying calls. Karen had answered a call from a young child playing with the telephone. She had called back and asked the child's parents not to allow the child to play with the phone. There had been a wrong number. Before becoming a 911 dispatcher, Karen might have thought it impossible to dial 911 as a wrong number, but now she knew that it was easy for someone to mistakenly dial 911 instead of 011—the access number for foreign telephone calls. Just a short time earlier, a teenage boy had asked her for a date before hanging up. He had not known that, with the enhanced 911 system, the dispatcher had a printout of not only his telephone number but also his address and the best way to get there. She had dispatched a Highbridge Falls Police patrol car to stop by at his house and have a little talk with his parents. Karen smiled as she wondered how long the boy would be grounded by his folks for that prank.

The phone rang. "What is your emergency?" Karen asked the 911 caller.

"I eet a mouse."

"You what?"

"I eet a mouse. I eet a mouse."

"Sir," Karen replied. "If you do not have an emergency, please do not dial 911." She disconnected the line.

Only a few seconds later the phone rang again. "What is your emergency?" Karen asked.

A man's hysterical voice said, "I eet a mouse. I eet a mouse."

Annoyed, Karen assumed her most authoritative tone of voice. "Sir," she barked. "This is an emergency line and we don't have time for your games. Please stop calling 911." She disconnected the call again.

Within less than a minute, the call came in again.

"What is your emergency?"

"I eet a mouse," the caller insisted.

Karen's patience was gone. She could see that the call

was coming in on a cellular phone and she was not able to trace the origin. "Sir, I don't care what you eat. People with real emergencies may not be able to reach us because of your prank. I can have you arrested for making a false report. Now please stop calling 911." Again she cut off the caller.

The line was silent for a couple of minutes. Then another call came in.

"What is your emergency?"

A weak voice replied. "We need help. We've been in an automobile accident."

Karen could see that this call too was coming from a cellular phone. "What is your location?" she asked.

"We're on Route 7, about a mile and a half north of the Highbridge Falls fire station."

"Are there any injuries?" Karen asked.

"My father seems to be all right, but I'm pinned in the car. I was stunned at first, but I think I'm okay. I'm not sure. There's blood and glass all over the place."

"Is there another car involved?"

"No. We hit a moose and it came through the windshield. I think it's dead, but it's on top of me. My dad tried calling you but he says you kept hanging up on him."

Oh, my God, Karen thought. The man who kept saying "I eet a mouse" and I thought he was a prankster. He hit a moose. "What is your name, sir?" Karen asked.

"It's Antoine. Antoine Chevreau."

"Antoine, I want you to stay on the phone with me until help arrives. They are on the way right now."

Within five minutes, Antoine, Eduard, and the moose were surrounded by police cars, fire engines, an ambulance, and a paramedic fly car. Except for a few lacerations

from broken glass, Eduard was uninjured and walked to
the ambulance. The paramedics were unable to examine
Antoine until the firefighters had cut the roof off the car
and carefully removed the dead moose. They were then
able to ascertain that most of the blood that covered
Antoine was from the animal. Antoine and his father
were transported by ambulance to the Highbridge Falls
Community Hospital where they were treated and
released a few hours later, but not before they were visited by a very contrite and apologetic 911 dispatcher
named Karen.

People in every profession have their crazy stories,
ones that you're sure couldn't have really happened. But
somehow they did.

A man called the emergency room at a local hospital
and told the nurse on duty that he had gotten his "pri-
vates" caught in his zipper and had suffered an abrasion.
He asked what he should do, and, as the nurse took a
breath to answer, he added, "It's the second time I got
stuck in these boot zippers," and hung up.

The ambulance was dispatched to an unconscious
person in a field about five minutes from headquarters.
As the ambulance rushed to the scene, lights flashing and
siren blaring, the radio sounded. "Police to all responding units, you can cancel your response. This scarecrow
isn't in need of any assistance."

The ambulance arrived at the scene of a possible heart
attack. The crew jumped out and rushed into the house. A

few moments later the fire engine arrived for an EMS assist. As they pulled up, they saw the ambulance driving away down the hill. Thinking that the call had been canceled, they started to drive away themselves, when they saw one of the EMTs walking from the residence. "We need the stretcher, guys," he yelled.

"But—" the engine driver said, then just pointed.

One of the firefighters and the EMT took off running after what was now assumed to be an empty ambulance, finally catching up to it after it had bounced over a set of railroad tracks, driven between several trees, and stopped, nose first, against a chain-link fence, going about thirty miles per hour.

The moral of the story: "Always set the emergency brake."

An ambulance was dispatched to a medical alert alarm at a residence on a quiet street outside of town. The crew arrived and tried the front door, with no success. One EMT walked around the house, looking for a way to make entry. When he arrived back at the front door, frustrated but still unable to gain entry, he found his partner halfway through a medium-size doggie door. Stuck for a moment, a foot in the seat of the pants propelled him through the opening. He opened the front door and the two searched the house but found no patient.

Moments later a car pulled up in front of the house. The driver, the owner of the residence, gave them his name and the EMTs introduced themselves. "Stupid thing was there for my mother who moved back to her own house months ago. I guess it went off by mistake. By the way, how did you get in?" the owner asked.

Only slightly chagrined, the EMTs explained. They

passed the house a few weeks later and found that the owner had dramatically reduced the size of the newly installed doggie door.

A crew was dispatched to a problem on the parkway. When they arrived they found that a police cruiser had pulled over an elderly man on a three-wheeled, battery-powered scooter. "A truck driver called this in," the officer said. "This guy was driving on the parkway."

The elderly man was quite confused, but finally managed to tell us that the adapter on his home oxygen setup had broken and he was driving to the medical supply store to get it fixed. Due to the lack of oxygen in his system, he became confused, took a wrong turn, and ended up on the parkway, unaware of his danger.

"Okay," the crew chief said, putting the elderly man on the rig's portable tank, "we'll take you over and help you get your tank fixed."

"What about my scooter?"

"You can't leave it here," the officer said.

They finally solved the problem by laying two long-boards as ramps from the ground to the back of the rig. With a little fancy maneuvering with both the scooter and the stretcher, they got both pieces of equipment into the back of the rig, with the patient in the front. The drive went smoothly until the EMT in the rear, trying to keep everything from rolling around in the back, found the horn of the scooter. He was a bit of a kid and the rest of the ride was quite noisy.

An ambulance was dispatched to a suicide attempt at the rear of a local convenience store. When the crew arrived they found a young man who had drunk a pint of Clorox.

"Why did you do this?" the police officer was asking.

"My wife left me and I lost my job."

"Why," the exasperated officer continued, "didn't you just get drunk like the rest of us would have done?"

"Oh," the young man said, "I don't drink alcohol. It's bad for you."

The crew arrived at the scene of an overturned vehicle. They found a very intoxicated man hanging from a rear seat belt, no sign of the driver. Worried that he or she might have been ejected from the vehicle, they asked the confused but seemingly uninjured man where the driver was.

"I'm the driver," he kept insisting from the rear seat.

When they finally pieced the story together, they discovered that he had had to blow his nose so he put the car into auto-pilot and got into the backseat. When he looked up, the car was going sideways so he snapped on his seat belt just in case. Auto-pilot, they ascertained, was cruise control.

In another case, a motor home stopped only inches from the edge of a steep dropoff. The driver had put on the "auto-pilot" and gone to use the bathroom while his family slept. "It's always worked before," he said.

Midafternoon on a hot, sunny Tuesday, a crew in Florida was called to the scene of a woman who had been shot in the head. Arriving at the car, parked in the parking lot of a local supermarket, they heard the woman screaming "I've been shot in the head. I heard the shot and I felt my brains."

They climbed into the hot car and examined the woman's head to find a lump of dough plastered against her hair. "How did this happen?" the crew chief asked.

"I went shopping, then ate a sandwich here in the car. I heard the shot. I've been shot."

The EMTs found no injury, then searched the car. Finally they found a can of refrigerator biscuits that had exploded in the Florida heat. It was several minutes before the woman believed that she hadn't been shot.

Nursing homes can be wonderful places. Occasionally they aren't.

At one, the crew arrived to find a woman in cardiac arrest. "Why isn't anyone doing CPR?" they asked as they began efforts to resuscitate the elderly woman.

"Oh, we can't do CPR," one of the nursing home employees said. "Our cards have expired."

A call came in from another nursing home. "CPR's in progress. Hurry." Another call came in moments later. "I'm . . . the . . . patient. Tell . . . them . . . to . . . stop . . . beating . . . on . . . my . . . chest."

Older people get lonely in the middle of the night, and occasionally, for want of anyone else to talk to, they dial 911.

It was about 11:00 P.M. and a crew responded to the residence of a sixty-five-year-old man who was complaining of chest pain. The crew arrived and were met at the door by the patient. He invited the two EMTs in and led them down a short hall into the living room. He sat down.

"What's your problem this evening?" one of the EMTs asked.

"I can't walk."

"But, sir. . . ." After a bit of questioning, they were able to establish that he wasn't really having any chest pain or serious difficulty walking. His only problem, he finally admitted, was that his legs felt weak.

"How long has this been going on?" the EMT continued.

The man stated that it had been like this for over a year.

"So why did you call us this evening?" the EMT asked, trying to maintain his patience.

"Well, I called my doctor's office and I got no answer. So I thought you might drive me over there."

"But, sir, it's almost midnight. Your doctor isn't in his office."

"Oh." He eventually refused any treatment or transport.

An ambulance arrived at a very rundown home in a rural area to transport a woman with severe abdominal pain. Suspecting several possible problems, the paramedic asked the woman whether she was sexually active.

"Not really," she said. "I just lie there."

A few years ago two EMTs were in the ambulance, having just come back from a call. They stopped at a large fresh fruit market to pick up some things for lunch. As he walked around at the rear of the store, one of the EMTs slipped in a puddle of water and went down very hard, striking the back of his head. He was unconscious for several moments and his partner, waiting in the rig, was unaware that anything had happened.

"I'm really all right," he assured the manager as he awoke. "I just need a minute to catch my breath."

"Don't worry, son," the manager said. "I called the ambulance."

At that moment the EMT's pager went off and he grimaced. "Unfortunately I am the ambulance crew today."

"You guys sure are fast," the manager said.

A woman put kerosene on her head to get rid of lice, then, with her hands still wet, she lit a cigarette. She got rid of the lice, and her hair. Fortunately she wasn't badly burned.

A crew arrived at the scene of an unknown medical emergency to be greeted by a naked man screaming, "She can't stop coming. She can't stop coming!"

They went into a back bedroom and found a woman, now recovering from a grand mal seizure, which had begun while she and the naked man were making love.

And an old EMS joke.

Two medics are discussing whether there is EMS in heaven. Finally, after a lot of wrangling, they decide that the first to die will come back and inform the other of what is up there. Unfortunately, one of the two is killed in an auto accident a few weeks later. He goes to St. Peter and asks about EMS. "I'll show you," St. Peter says, eager to show off heaven's facilities.

After a lengthy tour, the medic asks St. Peter for a favor. "I want to tell my buddy about your facility," he says. St. Peter agrees.

When he arrives at his house, his medic friend is surprised to see him, to say the least. "How is EMS in heaven?" he asks.

"I've got good news and bad news," the returnee says. "The good news is that they have state-of-the-art equipment of every kind up there. It's a medic's dream."

"What's the bad news?" the earthly medic asks.

"You've got the midnight-to-noon shift next Wednesday."

Chapter 9

Forty-three-year-old Jeff Garrett enjoyed working in his yard. He wasn't into flowers or vegetables, but he liked to keep the grass cut and the bushes and trees trimmed. The "back forty," as he referred to it, was a wooden section about fifty feet from the house. A few weeks earlier he had noticed several dead trees there. Worried that one might fall in a storm and damage his house, he decided to cut them down. "That way we can have wood for the fireplace all winter," he told his wife and children. "For free."

"Dear, isn't it dangerous?" his wife, Lorraine, asked. "I mean, you don't know anything about cutting down trees."

"Yeah, Dad. You're not Paul Bunyan, you know," Mike, his ten-year-old, said.

"Yeah, Dad," Andy, his six-year-old, chimed in.

"I'll get one of those books on outdoor fix-ups and it'll tell me all I have to know."

"Why don't we just hire someone?" Lorraine asked.

"That'll mean the wood won't be free. I can handle it."

"Can we have a really big fire?" Andy asked.

"We can have the biggest fire the fireplace can hold."

"Yippee," Andy cried.

Lorraine sighed. She knew Jeff well. Most of the time, if she just shut up, he forgot about plans like this and then, in a month or so, she'd hire a tree service to do the work.

But Jeff didn't forget. He got a book on tree pruning and found a section on how to take down small saplings. Bigger trees are just grown-up saplings, he reasoned, so it couldn't be too difficult. He read the book, then went to a local rental place and brought home a chain saw.

Knowing that Lorraine would object, he waited for a morning when she had gone out to run some errands, then took the chain saw to the backyard. The noise was deafening, but he made short work of a few shrubs and young trees that were in the way of the three larger trees he wanted to fell. He began with one that was already partially down and leaning against a larger, stronger tree. He reasoned it out well, and soon the branches were cut up for kindling and the trunk was lying on the ground in four large pieces.

"This isn't really hard," Jeff said, wiping his brow and refilling the gas tank of the saw. He straightened, rubbed his back, and stared at tree number two, a forty-foot-tall maple with an eighteen-inch-diameter trunk. It's half dead already and, Jeff reasoned, shouldn't be too much of a problem. Since it bordered the lawn area, he would cut it so that it fell onto the grass, angled away from the swing set and pool. He quickly cut a notch on one side, then one on the other. The book hadn't included any information on notching, but he'd seen it done in movies and it all seemed to make sense.

The tree, however, didn't fall as it did in the film he'd seen recently. It just stood there, laughing at him. He put both hands on the trunk and pushed with all his strength, but it remained standing. He took the saw and deepened one of the cuts until he heard the cracking sound that indicated that the tree was going over.

"Timber!" Jeff yelled, exhilarated that he had done it himself. But the tree listed in the wrong direction, ricocheted off a few larger trees, and, with much crashing and snapping, landed on Jeff's legs, pinning him to the ground and knocking him unconscious.

When he awoke, the pain was excruciating. The trunk lay across his lower legs and he couldn't feel his feet. He was lying on several sizable rocks and his back hurt. When he reached up and wiped his face, his hand came back bloody. "Oh, God. Oh, God." Then he started yelling.

Jeff had been on the ground for almost a half an hour before Lorraine finally returned from shopping. As she turned off the car engine she heard her husband's voice, now hoarse and almost crying. She ran across the backyard and, when she found him, knew immediately what had happened. "I'll call the fire department and the ambulance," she said, sprinting back to the house.

I was sitting at my computer, answering some of my e-mail, when the tones sounded. "Fairfax Police to Fairfax Ambulance."

After a pause, a voice answered. "Fairfax Ambulance is on. Go ahead, Fairfax Police."

"The ambulance is needed behind 223 Franklin for a man trapped under a tree," the police dispatcher said. "Is there a full crew at headquarters?"

"We have a driver and an attendant. Will you page out for an EMT please? 45–01 will be en route to 223 Franklin."

"10–4," the dispatcher said.

A man trapped under a tree? I dialed the phone. "Fairfax Police. Dispatcher Thomas."

"Mark, it's Joan Lloyd. I'll go to the scene."

"Great, Joan. Then the call's covered." The radio sounded again, announcing that fact to all ambulance corps members.

As I sprinted toward my car, I reprimanded myself. You promised. No calls today. You have work to do. I smiled. Yeah, I answered. But I'd rather do this. And this call sounds interesting.

When I arrived at the house on Franklin Road, two fire engines were already on location, but the ambulance hadn't arrived yet. I strode across the backyard and into the small wooded area at the rear of the property. Several firefighters waved me over and I knelt beside the injured man. He was in his forties, with a red plaid shirt and jeans. His face was pale and from his grimace I gathered he was in considerable pain. His face and arms were bloody and his lower body was hidden from view by the branches of a sizable tree. "What happened?" I asked. Then, as he looked up at me, I added, "Okay. Dumb question. It's pretty obvious. Where do you hurt the most?"

"I can't feel my feet and my legs hurt like hell."

"Can you move your toes?"

He hesitated. "No. Nothing."

"Okay, how about the rest of you? Did you black out when the tree fell?"

"I was out for a while. I have no idea how long. I must have gotten hit with a branch or something." He reached up and touched his forehead. "I'm cut and I'm scratched and bruised all over." He grabbed my shirt front and pulled me close. Softly he said, "And I'm scared shitless."

I took his hand. "I know. What I need right now is for you not to move your head or neck or anything." Tim Babbett ran up. Tim was in the middle of taking his EMT course and, although eager to help, he was not very experienced. "Tim," I said. "This is . . ." I turned to my patient. "What's your name?"

"Jeff Garrett."

"Tim, this is Jeff. I want you to hold stabilization and don't let him move his head or neck. Got that?"

"Sure," Tim said. He crouched above Jeff's head and placed a gloved palm against each side of his skull and extended his fingers along Jeff's face.

Fire Chief Paul Bradley walked up to us and put a tarpaulin over Jeff's torso from waist to neck. Then he handed me a helmet and put one on Tim's head. "We're going to cut away some of these branches," he said. "We'll try to keep everything clear of you but put this on, just in case."

"Okay, Chief." I put the helmet on then took a BP cuff and stethoscope from the crash kit Tim had brought. "Who's with you, Tim?"

"Fred's trying to get the rig in a spot that's out of the way but near enough so we don't have too long a carry." Fred Stevens is a tough, longtime member of the ambulance corps. He's a bit gruff with an odd sense of humor, but he's steady and solid.

"Jeff," I said, "it's going to get noisy, but these helmets and stuff are just for protection. Chief Bradley's the best. You met Tim, and my name's Joan, by the way."

Jeff smiled ruefully. "Glad to meet you, I guess, but I wish it were anywhere else."

I smiled back. "I'm sure you do and we do too."

While the sounds of sawing echoed through the yard, Tim leaned over Jeff to protect his face and I tried to take Jeff's vitals. I felt his pulse and counted his respirations, but when I placed the bell of the stethoscope against his inner arm and pumped the cuff to take a BP, I couldn't hear a thing. It takes a bit of quiet to be able to hear and in the din around us, there was no chance. So I found Jeff's radial pulse with my fingers and, as I inflated the cuff, I felt the pulse disappear. As I let the pressure down, I felt the pulse return. The reading on the gauge when I felt the first beat was a good measure of the systolic, or upper number, of Jeff's blood pressure. "I get 135 by palp," I said. I was glad that the number was well within normal limits for a man his age. "You've got a good strong pulse too, Jeff. You're doing well."

While firefighters sawed and cleared, I put a cervical collar around Jeff's neck to protect him from additional injury. Then I ran my hands over his head, neck, arms, and upper body. I found no swellings, deformities, indications of broken bones other than the head injury I knew about. The laceration I found just below his hairline was a bit swollen and tender to the touch, but the bleeding had stopped. I asked Jeff to take a deep breath and he assured me that there was no pain. His legs were the major problem, and there was little I could do while he was trapped beneath the tree trunk. From time to time, as the trunk shifted, Jeff screamed but he remained conscious and alert. Soon most of the major branches and all of the smaller ones were out of the way. The trunk, however, remained, keeping Jeff trapped.

As the sawing decreased, I finally got a clear look at what we were facing. The trunk of the tree, now about fifteen feet long, was resting across Jeff's legs, just below his knees. One end was about a foot and a half off the ground; the other had dug in and was just below ground level. Chief Bradley came up and filled us in. "Jeff, here's how it is. We can't saw any more of the trunk because we're afraid of putting extra pressure on your legs, nor can we just lift the high end because it's just too heavy and too unstable. So here's what we've decided. We're going to use our air bags to lift the tree off of you. It will take a few minutes but it's the best way."

Jeff was sweating and his skin was getting paler. I wanted the men to hurry, but I had worked with Chief Bradley many times and I was confident that he knew what he was doing.

"Air bags?" Jeff said. "Like in my car?"

"Not exactly. These are flat sort-of balloons. They're square, brightly colored, and capable of lifting a tremendous amount of weight." He pointed to a man carrying two eighteen-inch-square flat pieces of rubber, one bright red and the other hot yellow. "There they are. We're going to brace the high end of the trunk and then dig two small openings under the low end, put these in, and inflate them."

As we watched, two firefighters used small shovels to burrow beneath the trunk. Then the yellow air bag with a giant black X on the surface was wedged in one hole and the red bag in the other, with one-inch planking on both sides of each. Heavy cribbing of four-by-fours was placed under the raised end of the trunk, about six feet from Jeff's legs.

"Okay, Jeff," Chief Bradley said. "We're going to inflate these slowly and put additional cribbing in as the tree lifts. It might hurt but we have no choice."

"Okay," Jeff said, gritting his teeth. Tim continued to hold his head, and Fred and I moved back out of the way.

We walked over to a woman with tears streaming down her face who had been standing apart. "My name's Joan and this is Fred. We're with the ambulance."

"I'm Lorraine. Jeff's my husband."

I put an arm around her shoulder. "Chief Bradley and all his firefighters are the best. We've worked with them lots of times and I'm sure they'll have your husband free in no time." I hugged her. There was nothing more I could say, and platitudes were useless. To try to take her mind off of her husband's condition, I asked Fred, "Do you know how they blow those things up? I've never worked with the air bags before."

"Yeah. They use the air from the Scott packs," Fred said. "They really create a lot of pressure, more than enough to move that tree in just a few moments."

When everything was in place, the chief took control. "Listen to me," he yelled, and all other conversation ceased. "Up on yellow." A female firefighter turned a small knob and we heard a hissing sound. Slowly the yellow air bag began to inflate, raising the tree slightly. "Stop. Now up on red."

"Why are they using two?" I asked Fred.

"If it doesn't raise the tree enough, one bag will hold the tree in place while they crib and add another bag. You'll see."

As we watched, the chief alternately filled the yellow and red air bags until the low end of the trunk was about four inches off the ground. The chief looked at Jeff's legs carefully. "Not enough yet. Crib this, guys."

Several firefighters put wooden blocks beneath the lower end of the trunk and they deflated the yellow bag.

Someone brought a bright blue air bag and stacked it on top of the yellow. When the yellow was reinflated, the red was removed. "Okay. Just another few inches. Up on blue." Slowly the tree lifted another few inches, and as it did, Jeff screamed. Chief Bradley controlled the placement of one-, two-, and four-inch pieces of wood to support the trunk as it came still farther off the ground. When it was finally off Jeff's legs and stable, the chief waved us over. Fred and I had already agreed that the scoop stretcher was the best alternative for getting our patient out from under the tree with the least movement.

I moved to Jeff's feet and quickly cut up the front of his work pants. As I touched his legs, I found that they were severely deformed and uneven, but with little bleeding. "Jeff," I said loudly, "I'm going to try to take your shoes off. If I hurt you, let me know." I cut the laces of his work boots and slowly pulled them off, then cut his socks. I felt his feet and was amazed at how well the heavy boots had protected him. They were warm and I found a strong pulse in each. From the ankles down, there seemed to be no injuries. "Jeff," I said, squeezing his right big toe. "Can you feel this?"

"No," he said, now weeping openly.

"Can you move your feet at all?"

"No." He moaned.

"Okay. Just try to relax as best you can." Sometimes you say idiotic things just to make noise.

The scoop stretcher is made of two six-foot-long scissorslike metallic pieces that attach at both ends. Fred snapped the top end of the pieces together and we slid the now-vee-shaped contraption along either side of Jeff's body, with Tim still holding stabilization. Slowly we pushed the lower ends toward each other until they could be latched together.

There was little room to lift since the tree was still suspended over Jeff's body, so we slid the contraption, with Jeff on it, out, then lifted and placed him on the long backboard we had prepared earlier. We detached the scoop's sides and removed it, leaving Jeff on the backboard. While Fred and Tim immobilized Jeff's head, I placed one hand on either of his hips and pressed. "Does this hurt?" I asked.

"No," Jeff said. I touched his thighs, one at a time, and Jeff told me that they were all right. His knees seemed relatively undamaged too. The worst of the injury started in the middle of his lower legs. I could splint them, but I felt that the longboard he was lying on would do the job just as well. I folded a heavy blanket and placed it between his slightly separated legs and placed rolled-up towels on either side of his calves and ankles. I rechecked his pedal pulses and the neurological function in his feet and found everything unchanged. Then I asked several firefighters to lift the board carefully.

As they held the board off the ground, I took a roll of silver duct tape and wound it around and around Jeff's lower body, trying to apply even pressure rather than the concentrated pressure that tight separate straps would provide.

After about a dozen turns around the board and Jeff, I tore the tape. We strapped his upper body and taped his head in place. Fully packaged, he was now ready for transport.

"Thanks, guys," I said as the firefighters set the board on the stretcher and we strapped Jeff to it. "Great job!"

In the ambulance I took another set of vitals and was

surprised that he was still stable. With Jeff's wife in the passenger seat beside him, Fred drove slowly and carefully toward St. Luke's Trauma Center, fifteen minutes away. At every bump, Jeff screamed. "God, it hurts so much. You gotta stop the bouncing."

He must have some feeling in his legs, I thought, and for that reason I was glad he was in pain. But I didn't want to share my thoughts with my patient and possibly scare him more. "Jeff," I said. "We have two choices. We can go very slowly and try to eliminate the bumps, but that will take much longer to get you to the trauma center. If we go a bit more quickly, it might hurt more, but we'll get there faster. Which would you like?"

I find that giving the patient some sense of control often helps a situation. "Get there," Jeff hissed through gritted teeth. "You're right. I'll hang on."

With Jeff supplying information, I began writing up the PCR. About halfway down the parkway I said, "I'm going to call the trauma center and let them know we're coming. I want you to listen and be sure I get all the information correct. No secret messages. Okay?"

"Okay," he said, now a bit calmer.

I pressed the keys that would signal the trauma center that we had a message for them. "This is Fairfax 45–01 to St. Luke's ER."

"Go ahead, Fairfax."

"Be advised we are en route to your location with a forty-three-year-old male who was trapped beneath a fallen tree. He has crushing injuries to both lower legs, just beneath the knees, and a small head laceration. Patient states he was knocked unconscious for a short time. We have vitals as follows. Pulse 78 and strong, respirations 18 and regular, BP is 132 over 84 and has remained constant throughout the hour that it took to extricate him. Our ETA is seven minutes."

"We read you, Fairfax. We'll give you a room assignment on arrival."

"10–4. 45–01 is clear."

To keep Jeff as comfortable as we could, Fred did about forty miles an hour down the parkway, then slowed to about twenty through the hospital area. Once we were parked in the ambulance bay, we carefully lifted the stretcher from the rig and wheeled Jeff into the main trauma cubicle, where several staff members were ready for him. We finished our paperwork, put new linen on the stretcher, and, as we were ready to leave I stuck my head into Jeff's cubicle. "Good luck, Jeff," I said.

"Thanks for everything, Joan," he said. His wife looked at me and smiled weakly.

I thought about Jeff a lot for a while, then I moved on to new calls. It was almost six months later, and I was on line at the bank, when I ran into Jeff's wife. "I remember you," she said. "You were there when Jeff got hurt."

"Yes, I was," I said, remembering the woman instantly. "How is he?"

"Well, he's had six surgeries to put pins in his legs, but he's home now, on crutches with leg braces. It's tough on him and he gets lots of physical therapy. He'll never walk the way he used to, but they have hope that he'll eventually walk without even a cane."

"It must be a difficult time for you. How are you holding up?"

"I'm okay. But I'll tell you this. He's a lousy patient." She grinned at me. "But he's mine and I love him."

*   *   *

Most of the calls we respond to are simple and pretty routine. In most cases we move the patient to the ambulance and transport him or her to the hospital, giving what physical care is needed and a lot of psychological first aid. And most of the time, when we return home, we go on about our business unaffected. Most of the time . . . but not always.

"Fairfax Police to the ambulance corps. You're needed at a personal injury auto accident on Hunter's Hill Road near the bad curve. The caller stated that it seems serious."

By the time Stephanie DiMartino answered and asked the police to tone out for a driver or an EMT to respond to the scene, I was already in my car. "45–24 to base. I'm responding to the scene."

"10–4," Stephanie said. "We're on our way. Responding to Hunter's Hill Road for a PIAA. And put the helicopter on standby."

I arrived at almost the same time as the rig and together Stephanie, Sam Middleton, and I approached Officer Chuck Harding. "What's up?"

"She's pinned. I've got the fire department responding for extrication. Should we launch the chopper? The woman's screaming that she can't breathe."

"Yeah," Stephanie said. "Get them here ASAP."

"Can we get into the backseat?" I asked.

"The rear passenger side door is open," he said.

"Stephanie?" I asked.

"You get in and I'll work from out here and help with helicopter communications," she said.

"Okay," I said, heading for the rear door. As I walked up to the car I could hear the woman screaming. The car had hit a tree head on, slightly toward the driver's side. The front end was crushed, pushing the dashboard into the passenger compartment. The windshield was broken and the car's body was contorted. The rear door on the driver's side was jammed shut, but the one on the passenger side was opened partway so I slithered into the backseat, trying not to jiggle the car. I slid into the seat behind the driver and took her head between my palms. "I'm going to hold your head so it doesn't move," I told the terrified woman. "What hurts?"

"I can't breathe," she said. "My chest hurts real bad."

"Try to relax and take slow breaths. Does it hurt more when you take a deep breath?"

"Real bad. Get me out of here. Don't let me die."

At that moment I did something I rarely do. I promised her something I had no reason to believe I could deliver. "I won't let you die. I'm going to take good care of you. The fire department will be here in just a moment, and we'll have you free in a sec. What's your name?"

"Just get me out of here," she cried. I wondered just how much real breathing difficulty she could be having if she was still able to yell so loudly.

Stephanie stuck her head in through the open door and I said, "Regular collar and oxygen for now." She nodded and left. "Try to calm down," I told my patient, keeping my voice soft and level. "Breathe in and out slowly and try not to talk."

"I'm sorry. I'm so scared."

"I know. My name's Joan. What's yours?"

"Nancy."

"Nice to meet you, Nancy." Stephanie reached into the

car and put a regular-size cervical collar and the oxygen on the seat beside me. "Nancy, I need for you to hold real still while I put this collar around your neck. Okay?"

"I guess."

I quickly fastened the rigid plastic collar around Nancy's neck, then attached a non-rebreather mask to the oxygen cylinder. I opened the valve and held my finger over the release opening until the bag beneath the mask inflated with 100 percent oxygen. I placed the cylinder on the front seat beside her. "I'm going to put this over your face to help you breathe," I said, fitting the mask to Nancy's face and looping the elastic around her head. "Just breathe slowly and gently," I said.

Engine 44–31 arrived and pulled in front of the damaged car, effectively blocking off the road from oncoming traffic. Another engine, which arrived seconds later, took position behind us and blocked the road from the other direction.

"Here's what's going to happen, Nancy," I said. "The fire department is going to use the Hurst Tool to cut you out of here." I hate the term "jaws of life." It sounds really dramatic, but to a patient trapped inside of a vehicle, it also sounds scary. "We get a ringside seat."

"Just get me out. I can't breathe. I'm going to die." It's said that when a patient tells you she's going to die, believe it. In this case I wasn't at all sure. Her color was good and she was talking loudly and frequently.

"You're not going to die. I'm here with you and I won't let you die. Period." I watched as firefighters surrounded the car, discussing the pros and cons of various ways to get the vehicle open. Finally one firefighter hooked up the hydraulic hoses to the cutters of the jaws and approached, tool in hand.

"Hey," I yelled. "Can you get something to cover us up?"

"Sure thing," someone called. A firefighter handed me a spare helmet and then covered us both with a blanket.

"It's going to get very noisy in here and you'll hear lots of metal snapping," I told Nancy. "But these guys are really good and they know just how to do their job. We're just under this blanket for precaution."

"Don't let me die," she said again.

"Don't worry. I'm right here with you."

"I'm sorry. I'm scared. Am I going to die?"

I was spared the need to answer as the whine and throb of the Hurst Tool drowned out all other sounds. They efficiently removed the driver's side door but quickly discovered that the dashboard was pinning Nancy beneath it. "We'll have to roll this back," a firefighter, whose name I remembered was Elaine, said.

"That's a girl," Nancy said, sounding a bit calmer.

"Yeah, under all that turnout gear she certainly is. And she's terrific at what she does too."

Using chain and another attachment for the Hurst Tool, the firefighters lifted the dashboard off Nancy's lap. Then, with cutters, they severed the steering column and cut the brake and gas pedals to free her feet. I looked over her body as well as I could and saw no obvious injuries. Maybe all this will amount to nothing, I thought. A broken rib or two.

All in all, it had taken more than twenty-five minutes to get Nancy free of the entangling metal. "Great job, everybody," I said as they lifted the blanket off of us. "Okay, Nancy," I explained, "we're going to slide you onto a longboard and get you out of here." I looked around and saw that the helicopter had managed to land on the roadway, in an area with lawns on either side. "You're going to get to the hospital in grand style. The helicopter is waiting for you."

At that moment she reached over her head and grabbed onto the lapels of my jacket, pulling me against the back of her seat. "Don't let me die," she said. "Please don't let me die."

"You're not going to die. There are two flight nurses out there who aren't going to let that happen."

I let her hang onto me for a moment while Stephanie, Sam, and a few firefighters got the stretcher and board set up. Then I said, "You'll have to let go now."

"Can I hold your hand?"

"As soon as we get out of here you sure can."

I could feel her sobs as the fear consumed her. Quickly and efficiently we slid Nancy onto the long backboard and strapped and taped her down. I reached for her hand and she grabbed and squeezed. With a death grip on my fingers, she was carried to the helicopter's stretcher, where Sharon Blackstone and Carrie VanWyk were waiting.

"Hi, Joan, Stephanie. What's the story?" Carrie asked.

"I don't have much," I said. "Nancy and I were a bit busy under there. I do have a rapid carotid pulse, about 100, and respirations of 28 and shallow. I tried for a radial pulse as we were getting her out, but I couldn't get one with all the movement. And you folks were here so efficiently that I didn't have time to get much else. She's complaining of severe pain in her left ribs. She wasn't seat-belted and there was no air bag in the car. There was considerable invasion of the passenger compartment and the windshield was shattered."

"Okay," she said. "We'll take it from here." She

looked down at the woman who was now her patient. "Hi. You're Nancy and I'm Carrie. I see Joan and Stephanie have been taking good care of you."

"You're in good hands, Nancy," I said, still holding her hand. "Carrie and I have known each other since she was a member of the ambulance corps."

While I watched and Nancy held my hand, Carrie took a quick set of vitals and Sharon started an IV line in Nancy's right arm. Their eyes met and Carrie started a second line in her left. "Nancy, Joan can't go in the helicopter," Carrie told her. "There's just not enough room. I'm afraid you'll have to let go."

"Carrie and Sharon will take really good care of you," I said, and Nancy reluctantly let go of my hand.

As the pilot stood, Carrie, Sam, and two firefighters loaded Nancy into the back of the helicopter. "How are her vitals?" I asked Sharon as she quickly scooped up their equipment.

"Not good. She's got almost no blood pressure and at least a partial pneumo- or hemothorax." Air or blood was keeping Nancy's lungs from performing. Not good at all, I thought. "She's going down the tubes fast."

"Take good care of her," I said. I didn't tell her that I had promised Nancy she wouldn't die.

"We will," Sharon said.

And they tried, but I found out later that day that Nancy died on the operating table.

I felt awful. I had visions of her clinging to my lapels for days. Although I regretted promising her that she wouldn't die, I hoped that maybe it gave her some comfort. But I couldn't keep it from happening and, despite Ed's help and support, I remained very depressed.

* * *

Three nights later, in the middle of the night, the tones went off. "Additional manpower is needed for a rollover on the northbound parkway about two miles south of the Route 10 entrance. Any units responding, please call headquarters."

Great, I thought. Another call usually snapped me out of my bad mood so, as I pulled on my clothes, I called in. When I arrived at the accident on the median of the roadway, there were three groups of EMTs and fire-fighters, each I assumed, around a different patient. I went toward the smallest group, one beside a pickup truck, lying on its side. Linda Potemski was crouching over a man, partly in and partly out of the front wind-shield. The roof had been peeled back and there was a firefighter climbing around the man's legs. "Joan," Linda said. "They just cut him out. Can you hold the head while I get vitals?"

"Sure," I said, climbing around the twisted metal. I laid gloved palms against the man's head, noticing as I did that he was probably in his thirties, well dressed, well groomed, but reeking of alcohol. "What's your name, sir?"

"Barry." His breath was enough to knock me over.

"What's the problem?" I asked him.

"I fucking crashed my car," he spat at me.

"I understand that, sir," I said. "I was asking what hurts."

"My fucking leg," he said. "And those assholes who cut me out of this thing hurt me like hell."

"I'm sure they had no choice, and we'll be as careful as we can."

"I think he's got a femur fracture," Linda said, setting up the traction splint.

As I held his head, Linda and Fred Stevens, who had

also arrived in response to the page, applied the traction splint. "That should feel much better," I said as Linda tightened the mechanism.

"Yeah," Barry said. "I guess." I could tell by how his body had relaxed that it was more than "I guess."

When Linda was done, we quickly slid Barry onto a longboard, strapped and taped him down, and transferred him to the stretcher. "Need me to go along?" I asked.

"If you can, I'd love the help in the back," Linda said. "I can't seem to find much more than the broken femur, but his vitals aren't great."

"No problem." I climbed into the ambulance and rode to the hospital, holding the man's hand. Good, I thought, he's not doing too badly, and this will wash the taste of Nancy from my brain. Barry told us he was an accountant and had stopped for a few after going to a movie. A few, I thought. It was almost 3:00 A.M.

As we approached the emergency entrance of St. Luke's Trauma Center, Barry began to drift off, whether sleepy, unconscious, or just drunk it was hard to tell. But he didn't seem to be in serious condition. Good, I thought. He'll do okay.

He didn't. I ran into Linda in the supermarket the following afternoon. "He died," she said in amazement. "I was visiting a friend in the hospital and I checked in the ER. He had a broken femur and one of the bone ends had cut the femoral artery. He bled out into his thigh before they could even get him to surgery."

"Shit."

"Yeah. Shit."

It had been a bad week.

* * *

I responded to another call two days later. It had been such a bad week that I seriously considered not responding to any more calls—ever. Maybe I'm getting too old for this type of thing, I thought. There had been no pager calls for me to think about because there had been full crews at headquarters for the few calls that had come in since the rollover. Then I heard the police tone out. "A full crew is needed for a man lying in the grass beside Route 10, at the corner of Mill Street. Any available units please call police headquarters."

I heard Dave Hancock call in that he would pick up the rig and, before I could think better of it, I radioed in as the EMT, en route to the scene. This is probably nothing, I thought. Someone lying down, tired from walking into or home from town. The police will get there and we'll be canceled. But I'll go anyway. Maybe it will get me out of my funk.

I drove toward the call location, just a short distance from my condo. "Fairfax police to responding units. Officer on the scene says it's a boy who was hit by a car. He's requesting that you expedite."

Reflexively I put my green light on the top of my car and plugged the wire into the cigarette lighter socket. I arrived in moments, parked, grabbed my crash kit, and ran over to Officer Eileen Flynn, who was crouched on the grassy side of the guard rail beside the road holding head stabilization for the silent boy.

"What happened?" I asked.

Eileen answered. "He was waiting for a friend to pick him up and a car swerved to miss a deer. It crushed him against the guard rail and then flipped him over it onto the grass. You'd better check his legs, Joan."

"Is he conscious?"

"He's with us," Eileen said as I gazed down at the supine young man, whose eyes were closed and whose face was tight and pinched in pain.

I pulled a pair of heavy shears from my crash kit and cut up the front of the legs of the boy's jeans. I didn't like what I saw. There was little bleeding but severe deformation and swelling on both lower legs. I guessed that they both were at best broken, at worst crushed. "What's his name?"

"Billy," Eileen said. "He's eleven and being very brave, aren't you, Billy?"

I placed one hand on the top of each still-sneakered foot. "It's okay, Billy. I want you to wiggle your toes for me."

He did and the toes on both feet moved. "Good job," I said. "I'm going to take off your shoes now and I'll try not to hurt you." I cut up the front of both shoes, severing the laces, and then the sneakers slipped off easily. I grabbed the big toe on his right foot. "Which toe am I touching?"

"Big," he said through gritted teeth. From his demeanor, I knew he must be in a lot of pain.

I squeezed the baby toe on his left foot. "Which now?" I asked.

"Little. Other foot."

"That's great," I said. "Does anything hurt besides your legs? Did you hit your head when you got flipped?"

"No. Just legs."

"Any trouble breathing?"

"No," he said. "I'm in Little League."

I knew what he was thinking; he wouldn't be playing again for a long time.

"What position?" Eileen asked.

He took a deep breath and I could see his body relax a bit. Although his sentences were punctuated with hisses of pain, he said, "I'm a shortstop. You know Derek Jeter? He's the rookie with the Yankees. My dad took me to see him."

Bravo, Eileen, I thought. Get him to concentrate on anything but his legs.

The ambulance arrived soon after and we carefully logrolled Billy onto a longboard and, after fully immobilizing him, transferred him to the stretcher. Again one of my patients was in serious condition, en route to the trauma center.

At St. Luke's I did the paperwork while Dave put fresh linen on the stretcher. A doctor I knew reasonably well came out of Billy's room. "How is he?" I asked.

"I can't give you details," he said, "and the parents are on the way, but I can tell you that his legs are crushed. He'll be in surgery later today and it will take lots of physical therapy, but I think he'll walk again. Kids are pretty resilient."

"Thanks, Doctor," I said. I didn't ask about Little League.

It had been a very bad week.

My mind understood everything about the odds of getting three such bad ones in a row, but somehow I felt jinxed. Fortunately I have Ed. Over the days that followed we talked about all the silly calls we'd had, and Ed did his best to give me the support I needed. But my stomach didn't know whether I wanted to take any more calls.

In the end, I wasn't given a choice. The following

Sunday night, Ed and I were on duty and we got a call for a woman having difficulty breathing. Bob Fiorella was bringing the rig from headquarters. As we drove to the scene, I said, "Ed, you crew chief this one, will you?"

Knowing how I felt, he agreed. When we got to the scene, an elderly woman lay in bed. "I'm so sorry to call you out in the middle of the night like this," she said, "but I just couldn't seem to get my breath."

"Do you have a history of breathing problems?" Ed asked.

"Yes," she said, looking at me. "I smoked, you know." She reached out and took my hand. "Did you ever smoke, dear?"

I smiled at her. "Yes, many years ago," I said, amazed by her conversation despite her obvious respiratory problems. Her lips were slightly blue and her chest heaved with every breath. "You shouldn't try to talk. It must make it more difficult to catch your breath."

"It does." But she kept on talking. "It was really hard to stop smoking, you know."

"I know," I said.

"I'm really sorry to call you out. You're so good. You look very familiar. I think you were on the crew that picked me up when I broke my hips three years ago." She sighed. "But you people do so much good that I don't expect you to remember a silly old lady like me." I knew that I had never been in that house before, but what did it matter?

I held her hand while Ed took her vitals. Then, when Bob arrived, we put the woman, whose name we had learned was Velda Prince, on oxygen and shifted her onto the stretcher. "Thank you so much for coming out in the middle of the night."

"That's what we're here for," I said.

"Yeah," Bob chimed in. "That's why they pay us the big bucks."

"But you're volunteers," she said, then smiled. "Oh, you're joking with an old woman."

"I hate to ask a lady," Ed said in the ambulance as he was filling out the paperwork, "but how old are you?"

"I'm ninety-three come next November," she said.

She continued to talk, almost nonstop, all the way to Fairfax General. We wheeled her into an ER cubicle, and before we left she grabbed my hand. "Thank you again so much."

I squeezed her hand. "You're very welcome."

Maybe the week hadn't been all bad.

There's a line from a poem I read recently that says something like Show me a person who interrupts TV, family, tender moments / And I'll show you a volunteer. Well . . .

Ed and I had finished dinner and were enjoying a "tender moment" when the pagers went off. In the seconds between the tones and the announcement from the dispatcher, Ed looked at me and I looked at him and we burst out laughing. Timing is everything, and the "tender moment" was totally interrupted.

"GKL–642, Fairfax Police to all home units. A full crew is needed for a PIAA on the parkway, south of the Route 10 entrance. Any available unit please call in."

Since the moment was ruined anyway, I looked at Ed and raised an eyebrow. "Sure," he answered, reaching for the phone and dialing. "Ed Herman and Joan Lloyd will respond directly to the scene," I heard Ed say as I quickly put my clothes on. When Ed was dressed, we rushed out of the house and drove toward the parkway.

When we arrived at the accident scene, we saw a car, its driver's side against the guard rail, its front windshield pushed out on the passenger side. The vehicle was already surrounded by fire and police personnel.

"What's the situation?" Ed asked.

"The man in the passenger seat is the only one injured," the officer said.

"Want me to hold head stabilization?" I asked Ed. When we arrive at the scene together, whoever asks the first question usually assumes the duties of crew chief, so in this case, Ed was in charge.

"Sure," he told me, so, with as little movement to the vehicle as possible, I climbed into the backseat of the small black car. "Okay, sir," I said, "I'm going to hold your head to keep you from moving. It's all precautionary."

"What happened?" Ed asked, leaning in through the window.

"I don't really know what happened," the injured man said. "The air bag hit me in the face."

I looked around as best as I could. There was blood all over the man's face and his eyes were swollen. The passenger side of the front window was pushed outward.

"Were you wearing a seat belt?" Ed asked.

"Yes."

I guessed the damage to the window had been caused by the pressure of the deploying air bag. The victim was a large man, probably almost three hundred pounds, and he had the front seat as far forward as he could. There had been so little room between the man and the dash-board that the air bag had had nowhere to go.

I looked over and saw that the driver was stuck in his seat between the injured passenger and the door, held closed by the guard rail. One of the rear passengers had climbed out, but the woman behind the driver was still in her seat. I quickly checked again and the driver denied any injury. "I just can't get out of here until they move George."

"And you, ma'am?"

"I'm fine," the woman said, patting the injured man on the shoulder. "He's my husband. Forty-seven years."

I smiled and nodded. Since I could communicate better with our patient than Ed could, I began a verbal assess-ment. "Sir," I said as Ed held the man's wrist to take a quick pulse, "my name's Joan and that's Ed who's got your wrist. And you're George?"

"Yeah. George McDermott," he said.

"Okay, George, where do you hurt besides your face?"

"I think the rest of me's okay," he said. "I'm a bit shaky."

"Of course you are," I continued. "Can you take a deep breath for me?" When he did, seemingly without pain, I continued, "Anything hurt now? Ribs, back, neck?"

"No," he said. "Just my eyes."

"Do the eyes themselves hurt, or around them?"

"My eyes don't really hurt, but it's all around them. And my face is bleeding."

"We'll take care of that in a minute. Do your fingers and toes wiggle?" I could see him move his hands and, since it was dark, I assumed he was trying his toes.

"Yup. Everything wiggles."

"That's great," I said.

"Forty-seven years," his wife mumbled. "We've never had anything like this before."

Ed wrapped a blood pressure cuff around the man's upper arm and began to take his BP. "I'm glad you haven't and I hope you never do again," I said. "Sir, do you have any medical history?"

"Marie?"

His wife said, "Nothing. In forty-seven years, nothing. Actually in seventy-one years that he's been alive there's been nothing wrong with him."

"I wasn't alive until I met you," George said.

"What a nice thing to say," I said, smiling. "So I assume you don't take any medicine on a regular basis?"

"Nope," he said.

"And how's your vision? Any double vision or blurriness?"

"Yeah," he said. "My left eye's a bit foggy."

"We'll get you out of here and then check your eyes." I looked at Ed as we heard the siren of the approaching ambulance. "The ambulance is here and we can get a collar around your neck and then get you out of this car." To the driver and George's wife, I said, "You two sure you're all right? Nothing bothering you now that you've calmed down a bit?"

"I'm fine," the driver said.

"Take care of George," the man's wife said.

"Ma'am, that's not what I asked. I want to know that you're all right. We'll take care of George just fine. I need to know how you are."

She hesitated, then said, "I'm okay. Really." She held up her hands. "See? Everything wiggles just like you said."

"Good. Everyone was wearing seat belts?"

"Yes," the driver said. "But the air bag. It hurt George's face. Isn't it supposed to help?"

"It did. Think about what would have happened without it. The seat belt stopped him somewhat, but his neck would have snapped and who knows whether he would have slid into the dashboard without it."

"Okay," Ed said, easing the passenger door open. "We're going to put a collar around your neck to protect you. It won't be comfortable, but that's not why it's there. It's to support your neck and to remind you not to move." As he slipped the end of the cervical collar between George's neck and the headrest, he continued, "Your vitals are good, your lungs are clear. I think your facial injuries are the only problem right now. We'll take you to the hospital where they can examine you." He fastened the Velcro to secure the collar.

"KED?" I asked, wondering whether we would use the heavy slatted jacket to immobilize the man's head, neck, and back.

Ed looked at the driver. "Can you open your door?" he asked.

The driver looked out his window. "No. I'm pressed up against the guard rail."

"Okay, then we'll have to just take him out on a board."

"What does that mean?" Marie asked.

"In order to get a KED on properly it needs to be positioned correctly, and that's just about impossible to do without someone who knows how on each side. So, since we can't get at George's other side, we'll take him out on a long backboard directly."

"Oh," she said, and sighed.

"He'll be fine," I said, trying to reassure her.

"I'm okay, Marie," George said.

We quickly transferred George to a long backboard, strapped him down, immobilized his head, and put him on the ambulance stretcher. In the rig, Ed checked his eyes with a penlight, then asked, "Do they hurt?"

"A little. They feel gritty and scratchy."

"It's probably from the dusty material that comes out when the air bag is deployed," Ed explained. "I'm going to cover them with a little gauze to protect them."

"Dear," Marie's voice called from the seat beside Nick Abrams, our driver, "I'm here in front. I'm going with you." Then under her breath I heard her say again, "Forty-seven years and nothing like this has ever happened before."

Both of George's eyes were very swollen, as was the area around them. "How about something cold on your face?" Ed asked.

I got a cold pack from the cabinet and smashed my fist into it until the inner container ruptured and combined the two chemicals. As the plastic bag got cold I covered George's eyes and orbits with four-by-fours, then placed the cold pack on top, holding it to lessen the pressure.

George sighed. "That feels nice," he said.

"Wonderful," I said. "It's always good to know that what we do helps."

We transported our patient to FGH and turned care over to the staff. I guided his wife to the admissions area so she could give all the pertinent insurance details to the receptionist.

As we were leaving, my thoughts turned to the "tender moment" Ed and I had been sharing. I winked at him and he winked back.

As we were returning to headquarters, the police dispatcher's voice came through our radio. "Fairfax Police to Fairfax Ambulance."

"45–01 on."

"Take a call for a woman who fainted at the A&P."

"Responding," Nick said into the mike.

I groaned and looked at Ed, who rolled his eyes. Nick flipped on the siren and we sped toward the supermarket. When we arrived we were directed to line 2, where we found a middle-age woman seated on the floor. "I'm fine now," she said quickly. "I really don't need an ambulance. I just felt a little light-headed, so I sat down."

"Good thinking," I said, sitting down next to her. "My mother always said that no one was ever injured from passing out. It's hitting the ground that does the damage. How do you feel now?"

"I'm okay. I didn't have dinner and I sometimes have trouble with my blood sugar." A young man in a green A&P jacket handed the woman a Milky Way. "Thanks," she said. "This will fix everything." She tore off the wrapper and took a tremendous bite.

"Why don't you let us at least take your pulse and blood pressure?"

"If you need to," she mumbled, her mouth full of candy.

Ed quickly took a set of vitals. "You seem just fine," he said. "Your pulse is a bit fast but your blood pressure is normal: 114 over 76."

"Good," the woman said, taking another giant bite.

"Let's get your name and address and then we'll see how you feel." Ed efficiently took down the woman's name, address, medical history, and the other information necessary for our prehospital care report. By the time he finished, she had eaten the entire candy bar and was starting on a bag of M&Ms with almonds.

She heaved a great sigh. "Much better now," she said. "The candy will get me going and the nuts in the M&Ms will keep me until I get home and eat something. It was a dumb thing to do."

"Well, we can take you over to the hospital and let them examine you," Ed said.

"Not a chance. I'm really fine now."

"Why don't you see how you feel when you stand up?"

She got to her feet and, after a bit of initial unsteadiness, she seemed fine.

Ed took her wrist and felt her pulse. "It's much better now. If you're sure. . . ."

"I'm sure." She signed our form and we left. On our way back to headquarters, we grinned at each other. Maybe we would be able to recapture our "tender moment," but as volunteers, we knew we might be interrupted at any time. Fortunately, we do our EMS work together so we understand the adrenaline rush when the tones go off. I wonder how folks do this when their spouse isn't involved. Oh, well, Ed and I are lucky to have each other.

Chapter 10

It was a steamy August morning. Twelve-year-old Rosa Chen and two of her friends had decided to go swimming at the gorge, where the Fairfax River continued toward the sea below the reservoir spillway. Since both of Rosa's parents worked, she was on her own for most of the summer. Rosa had her parents' permission to swim at the gorge, but as to swinging on the rope ... well, that was a different matter. A rope had been tied to the branch of an old tree and for as long as anyone could remember local kids had used it to swing themselves out from the steep slope of the gorge. Then they would let go and drop about thirty feet into the river.

Rosa's best friend, Sandy, was the first to grab the rope. Gracefully she swung out and, with a shriek of delight, released her hold and plunged into the cold, deep water. Rosa watched apprehensively. Janet went next and, with a seemingly effortless swing, splashed into the icy water. "Go ahead," Sandy yelled. "It's easy."

Rosa wasn't at all certain that she wanted to do it. Sure, it looked like a lot of fun, but, even though Rosa had always been very adventurous and athletic, her body had changed so much in recent months that she wasn't at all comfortable with her ability to swing her weight around. Also, although her father had given her permission to use the rope, her mother had said "Absolutely not," and Rosa knew the rule. She had to have the okay from both parents for something like that.

"Go ahead, Rosa," Janet now joined in, as Sandy, who had climbed back up the slope, held the rope out to her. "Don't chicken out."

Oh, well, Rosa thought, it looked really easy when Sandy and Janet did it, and my mother won't find out. Rosa grabbed the rope and started her swing, but as soon as her feet left the ground she knew she was in trouble. She desperately tried to hold on to the wet, slippery rope even as she felt it slip through her fingers. Suddenly she was falling through space and watching the ground coming to meet her.

Joan and I were on duty with Stephanie DiMartino at FVAC headquarters when the klaxon sounded. "GKL–642 Fairfax Police to Fairfax Ambulance."

Stephanie keyed the mike. "FVAC on. Go ahead, Fairfax Police."

"Respond the ambulance to the swimming area at the gorge. We have a report of a child injured in a fall."

"10–4, Fairfax Police. We're on our way."

"You're en route at 11:04. Fairfax Police clear."

As we pulled up above the gorge, I could see Police Officer Will McAndrews and a small group of kids clustered around a girl who appeared to be in her early teens. She was wearing a bathing suit with a pair of old jeans, cut off at the knee, over it, and there were thin trails of blood trickling down her wet shins. She was sitting on a railing at the side of the road, screaming "She'll kill me. She'll kill me."

I looked at Joan. "This looks like a job for supermom."

"What's the story?" she asked Will.

"A very lucky twelve-year-old who was swinging on the rope and fell about ten feet onto the rocks at the edge of the river," Will replied.

I looked down the gorge at the river, about fifty feet below. "How did she get back up to the road?" I asked.

"Oh, she climbed back up by herself. She doesn't seem to have any serious injuries."

"She'll kill me. She'll kill me," the girl continued to cry.

Joan turned to one of the other girls in the group. "What's her name?" she asked.

"It's Rosa," one of the girls replied.

"Rosa," Joan said, taking the girl's head in her hands, as much to get her attention as anything else. "I want you to calm down and tell me where you're hurt."

"My legs," the girl cried, "but she'll kill me."

"Do you have any pain in your neck or back?" Joan asked.

"She's gonna kill me," Rosa yelled.

"Who's gonna kill you?" Joan asked.

"My mom. My mom. She told me not to do it. She's gonna kill me."

"Rosa, your mom isn't going to kill you. She'll be happy that you're not badly hurt. Now I need you to tell me whether your neck or back hurts," Joan said calmly.

"No, just my legs," Rosa replied.

"Okay," Joan said. "This is Ed. He's going to examine you. I want you to tell him if anything hurts."

"All right." Rosa sniffled, beginning to calm down.

I carefully palpated Rosa's head, neck, and back, while Joan held head stabilization. There was no bleeding, swelling, deformity, discoloration, or point tenderness anywhere.

"Rosa," I said. "I'm going to have to cut the bottoms of your pants so I can examine your legs."

"But they're my favorite jeans," she protested.

"Well, if you'd rather, we could try to get them off you without cutting them. . . ."

Rosa looked down at her lower legs, bruised and scraped in a few places from the rocks. It was obvious that she realized how difficult it would be to try to maneuver the heavy, wet denim over them. "No, you can cut them," she said, obviously not pleased with the alternative.

A complete body survey showed discoloration and point tenderness in both knees and Rosa's left shin. There were a couple of small lacerations on her shins and on the top of her right foot. "I don't think we need to board and collar her," I said to Joan. "There's no indication of head or spinal injury. And after her climb up the slope, I don't see any point in splinting her legs. There's no indication of any fracture. I'll just dress those lacerations and we can get her into the ambulance. I don't think you have to continue to hold head stabilization."

Rosa looked down at her foot. "Oh my God, I'm bleeding," she yelled.

"It's just a couple of small cuts," I assured her. "I'm just going to dress and bandage them to keep them clean."

"I don't want any stitches," Rosa screamed.

"They are very small cuts," I said. "I don't think that you will need any stitches."

"Are you sure?"

"No. I'm not a doctor, Rosa. I can't give you a guarantee. But I'm pretty sure."

"Don't put alcohol on them," Rosa yelled.

"I'm not going to put anything on the cuts except a sterile dressing," I replied.

"But they will use alcohol to clean them at the hospital, right?" Rosa said, her voice rising.

"Rosa, listen to me," Joan said. "They won't do anything at the hospital until your mother arrives. And then they won't do anything that you and your mother don't agree to."

"Tell them not to put alcohol on my foot."

"You can tell them yourself at the hospital. But not by yelling like you're doing now. If you discuss it with them calmly, like an adult, they will be responsive. If you scream at them, they'll treat you like a child."

While I dressed and bandaged Rosa's shin and foot and Joan continued talking to the girl, Will and Stephanie brought over the stretcher. We quickly got Rosa into the ambulance, where she again started to become agitated. "If my leg's broken they're going to have to set it. It's gonna hurt like it did when they set my broken arm."

"They will probably take X rays to make sure, Rosa," I said, "but I don't think you have any broken bones."

"You've had fractures before?" Joan asked.

"Yeah, I broke my arm three times," Rosa replied.

"Are you a bit of a tomboy?" Joan asked.

"Yeah. I guess," Rosa said with a small smile.

"Do your parents work nearby?" Joan asked.

"My dad works in the city but my mom works in Prescott. The police called her. She's gonna come to the hospital. She's gonna kill me." Rosa was starting to cry again.

I picked up the PCR box and started to fill out the report. "I need your full name, Rosa," I said.

"It's Rosa Chen."

"Chen?" I repeated. "And your mother works in Prescott?"

"Yeah. She's gonna kill me. I wasn't allowed to swing on the rope."

Joan and I glanced at each other. "Is your mom a paramedic?" I asked.

"Yeah. She works for the Prescott Fire Department."

"You're Amy's kid?" Joan asked.

"Yeah. Amy Chen. That's my mom. And she's gonna kill me."

It was all I could do not to laugh. Amy was one of the gentlest, nicest people I knew. We had worked many calls together in the Prescott Rescue Squad. She was one of Prescott's finest paramedics.

"Rosa," I said, "I've known your mom for years. I may not be able to promise you that the hospital people won't put alcohol on your cut or that you don't have a fracture, but I can promise you absolutely that your mom won't kill you."

Having been alerted about her daughter's accident by radio, Amy was waiting for us when we pulled into the emergency bay of Fairfax General. "She's just fine," I said to Amy as we wheeled Rosa into the ER. "She's got some bumps and bruises and a couple of minor lacerations, but that seems to be all."

Amy looked at Rosa and snapped, "Who cut your pants?"

"They did, Mom," Rosa said defensively. "I didn't want them to, but they did."

"Well, I'm gonna put Joan and Ed in for a commendation," Amy said, suddenly grinning. "I've been wanting to get rid of those ugly jeans for a long time."

"Are you mad?" Rosa asked, her voice tiny.

"I'm not happy that you disobeyed, but I'm glad you're okay. We'll talk about the details later."

We left the two in a small side cubicle.

By the time we returned to headquarters, I was feeling confident of my ability to deal with adolescent girls. Our duty shift was over and no one had signed on for the afternoon shift, so the police would have to set off the pagers if a call came in. Joan had gone home to wait for the cable TV repairman and I decided to stop for gas. I was heading north on Route 10 when the next call came in. "GKL–642 to all pagers and home monitors. A full crew is needed for a child struck by a car on Route 10, in front of Angela's Pizza."

I grabbed the portable radio from the seat next to me. "45–22 to GKL–642. I'm about zero-one minutes from the scene. I'll proceed as the EMT. Have a driver and attendant meet me there with the rig."

"10–4, 45–22."

As I proceeded to the accident scene I could again hear the pager tones on my portable radio. "GKL–642 to all pagers and home monitors. A driver and attendant are still needed for a child struck by a car. Will a driver and an attendant please call in."

Less than a minute later, I pulled over behind a Fairfax patrol car, grabbed my stethoscope and small roll of duct tape, and trotted over to where Officers Merve Berkowitz and Eileen Flynn were struggling with a young girl who was shrieking and flailing her arms and legs. Joan thinks that my wearing a stethoscope draped around my neck is an affectation. She's right, it is. But it's also an instant means of identification and saves me the time and trouble of ever having to explain who I am at an emergency medical scene. Occasionally I even use the stethoscope. Duct tape, on the other hand, is no affectation. It is one of the most useful pieces of equipment that an EMT can carry. No other means of immobilization, including the most expensive devices, is as fast and effective as plain, ordinary duct tape.

Seeing that, despite their best efforts, Eileen and Merve were not able to immobilize the girl effectively, I grabbed her head while they tried to hold her arms and body still. I looked at Eileen. "What happened?" I asked.

"Her friend, over there"—Eileen nodded toward a weeping girl at the side of the road—"says that they were trying to cross the highway. This girl ran out directly into the path of an oncoming car. According to her friend she was thrown about twenty feet."

I struggled to hold the girl's head as she cried and fought our efforts to restrain her. "Terri, calm down," Eileen yelled. "We're just trying to help you."

The girl showed no sign of having heard, and continued to scream and struggle.

"Do you know the extent of her injuries?" I asked.

"There doesn't seem to be any bleeding, but all we've really been able to do is try to restrain her so she doesn't hurt herself further. She was just flopping around in the road when we got here," Eileen said.

"Terri, can you tell me where you're hurt?" I yelled.

The girl continued to shriek and struggle, and it took all my strength to hold her head still. I looked at as much of her body as was visible. There were no obvious deformities and there was no bleeding. Her left temple, close to where my hand was pressed against her head, had a large abrasion, but there was no swelling. The wound looked more like road rash than a serious head injury, and her clothing did not appear to be torn. "Does anyone know how old she is?" I asked.

"Her friend says she's twelve," Eileen said.

"Amazing. She's so tiny she looks about eight."

Merve grabbed an arm that had wriggled out of his grasp. "But with the strength of an eighteen-year-old body builder," he added.

Eileen, Merve, and I could do nothing further until the ambulance arrived. At last we heard the wail of the siren and the ambulance pulled up. Dave Hancock and Pam Kovacs came over. "What do you need, Ed?" Pam asked.

I looked at our diminutive patient. "Get a pede collar, and oxygen. And let's try the pede board."

The pediatric board, also known as a "papoose," is a very effective device that uses Velcro straps to completely immobilize a child. Dave and Pam brought over the equipment, but Terri struggled so much when they attempted to apply the pediatric cervical collar that I decided that we were doing more harm than good. "Let's just get her on the pede board," I suggested. "We can use a blanket roll to immobilize her head."

Getting her on the pede board was not going to be easy either. Soon everyone was feeling frustrated and was yelling at Terri above her screams.

"Terri, calm down."

"Terri, we're not going to hurt you."

"Terri, stop fighting us."

"Terri, stop screaming."

Suddenly I yelled as loud as I could. "Hey."

Everyone except Terri stopped talking and looked at me. "Everyone's yelling at her," I said. "How about letting me be the only one talking to her? Maybe I can calm her down."

I lowered my voice and, despite her continued shrieking, began to talk to her calmly. "Terri," I said. "We're only holding you so hard because you're fighting us. If you stop trying to move your head, I won't have to hold it so tightly."

I continued talking to the girl in a low voice and in a few moments she began to calm. Thinking that my talking to her was being successful, I encouraged her. "That's very good, Terri. You're doing fine."

Suddenly Terri closed her eyes and went completely limp. "Terri," I said.

There was no response. Terri appeared to be unconscious. I pinched her arm and there was no reaction. Now I was suddenly much more concerned about my patient. Her combative behavior and her current lack of responsiveness were indications of serious head trauma and possible brain damage.

We quickly got a cervical collar around Terri's neck and placed an oxygen mask over her face. Then we slid the pediatric board under her but the Velcro straps would not close. Terri was just a bit too big for it. "Okay, get a long backboard, head blocks, and spider straps. Let's board her and get her to the hospital." We had just gotten her onto the longboard and were about to fasten the restraining spider straps when, with a shriek, Terri yanked her arm free, reached up to her neck, and tore the heavy-plastic cervical collar in half, then pulled the oxygen mask from her face. There was now no way that we were going to be able to use the spider straps to secure the girl to the longboard without spending a lot of time doing it.

"Dave," I yelled, struggling again to maintain head stabilization. "Reach into my pocket and take the roll of duct tape. Let's just tape her to the backboard and get her to the hospital."

Dave, Merve, and Eileen lifted the board and I wrapped the duct tape around and around Terri's body and the board, effectively immobilizing her. Within a few moments we were able to transport her to Fairfax General.

Terri continued to alternate between screaming and unconsciousness while en route to the hospital. Although I talked to her continually, she gave no indication that she heard me at any time. At the hospital, with some grumbling, the ER staff removed the duct tape and Terri was given medication to calm her. Dr. Margolis asked me to stay and maintain manual head stabilization while he examined the girl and a nurse started IV lines in both arms.

I was still holding Terri's head when her mother arrived, obviously upset but not frantic. "Terri has two older brothers who have been to the emergency room many times," she said. "I'm kind of used to this. Terri, it's all right. I'm here, baby," she said quietly into her daughter's ear.

Terri's eyes were wide open and she yelled, "Mom, where are you?"

Terri's mother, who was standing on the girl's right side, next to the examination table, replied, "I'm right here, baby."

"I can't see you," Terri cried. "Why don't you come where I can see you?"

"But I'm right here next to you," she said, glancing at Dr. Margolis in alarm.

Dr. Margolis held a penlight out in front of Terri. "I want you to look at this light, Terri," he said. He moved the light from right to left and from left to right while shining it in Terri's eyes. I could see that Terri was able to follow the light to the left but not to the right where her mother stood. I had a hollow feeling in my gut. Terri's inability to track to the right was another indication of brain damage.

"Why can't she see me?" Terri's mother asked Dr. Margolis, obviously terrified.

"We won't know anything until we send her upstairs for a CAT scan," Dr. Margolis replied somberly. It was obvious that he feared the worst.

The rest of the day was a washout for me. I couldn't work and I couldn't get Terri out of my mind. I was certain that she had suffered serious brain trauma, and I just hoped that she would survive her head injury without too much disability. We should have been able to immobilize her more quickly, I thought. We should have gotten oxygen on her sooner and kept it there somehow. At dinnertime I wasn't very hungry, and that evening I decided to drive over to Fairfax General to see if I could find out how the girl was doing. As I pulled into the emergency room parking lot, I couldn't believe my eyes. Terri and her mother were walking out of the hospital. Terri's mother saw me get out of the car and waved to me. I walked over and looked at the girl incredulously. "I came over to see how Terri was doing," I said.

"Oh, she's just fine," the mother said. "She snapped out of it about an hour after you left. The CAT scan and all the other tests were negative. The doctor said she had a concussion that caused her temporary visual problem, but, except for a scrape on her head and a bruised knee, she has no other injuries. They kept her in the emergency room all afternoon for observation but decided that there was no point in admitting her. I'm supposed to keep an eye on her for forty-eight hours, but I'm sure she's all right."

Terri's mother turned to her daughter. "Terri, this is one of the people who took care of you in the ambulance. This man held your head all the way to the hospital."

Terri looked at me, obviously unimpressed. "Hi," she said, then turned to her mother. "Hey, Mom, can we pick up some KFC for dinner? I'm starving."

"Sure, baby," her mother said. "Let's go." She turned to me. "Thanks for everything."

As I watched them walk away, I felt confused, enormously relieved, and amazed at the incredible good fortune that had allowed two teenage girls, Rosa and Terri, to continue with their lives after coming so close to permanent injury or death.

Someone once said that childhood was just "life, with training wheels." I hoped the training wheels would be enough to keep these two from further harm.

I was hard at work at my computer. Unavoidable Christmas music filled the airwaves. Lord, I was tired of "Little Drummer Boy" and "White Christmas."

My Prescott pager sounded. "GVK–861 to all home units. A full crew is needed Park Manor for a man down."

It was Christmas morning and I knew no one would want to respond. Let them stay home with their families, I thought, picking up the phone. Park Manor is a residence facility for the lonely, unloved, and those who are euphemistically described as "less fortunate." Many of the residents are mentally ill or physically handicapped, and they spend most of their time standing around in the lobby or wandering the neighborhood, occasionally getting hit by cars. The facility is funded by some governmental organization, but the funding is constantly being cut so Park Manor is shabby and poorly staffed. The overworked employees usually try to be helpful and pleasant; the residents are distant and vague.

I picked up the phone and pressed the speed dial. "It's Ed," I said to the dispatcher. "I'll respond to headquarters."

"Come on in, Ed. Brenda Frost is responding and Max called in to drive."

"On my way," I said.

The drive to the firehouse is short but the rig was already waiting for me, red lights flashing. I jumped into the back and yelled "Hi" to Brenda and Max.

"Amy's on this morning," Brenda said, referring to Paramedic Amy Chen. "She's responding from the hospital with a short delay." That meant we'd be there before she would. "She just came in with a woman who burned herself on grease, basting her Christmas turkey."

I smiled and shook my head. Holidays! Okay, I grumbled to myself, I'm starting to sound like Ebenezer Scrooge. Get over it.

We pulled into the parking area in front of the manor, stopped behind the fire engine, and climbed out. I carried the trauma bag and Brenda grabbed the oxygen duffel. We opened the front door and were assaulted by heat and the smell of stale air and not very carefully washed bodies. Several people stood around the lobby, some lined up at the desk for their morning medication. All moved slowly and looked slightly vacant.

The walls hadn't been painted for several years but the dull, institutional beige had been covered with Christmas decorations. Garlands of colored paper, tinsel, hand-colored paper wreaths, bright blue plastic rope and sprays of green plastic pine covered most of the surfaces. At least they try, I said to myself.

Several people pointed toward the rec room, a large, sparsely furnished area with a television and several old Formica tables with cracked plastic chairs. With Max just behind pulling the stretcher, Brenda and I strode through the large doors.

Pete Antonio, the engine driver, crouched beside a man of undetermined years who lay sprawled on the floor. The man's eyes were open and he looked as if he had last shaved about a week before. "I just got here," Pete said, immediately moving to one side of the dimly lit room. He was new and young, and although he was an EMT he looked overwhelmed.

I pressed my gloved fingers against the man's carotid artery. "No pulse." I turned to a woman in a pair of worn jeans who looked like she might be staff, not a resident. "Who found him, when and where?"

"I found him," she said. "I was handing out meds and he said he had to go to the bathroom. When he didn't come back in a few minutes I went to look. I found him on the bathroom floor and dragged him out here. That was when I called 911, about maybe ten minutes ago."

"He's still warm," I said, knowing that there was not much chance to bring him back. Unless CPR is begun within five minutes there's little hope. "Let's do it."

Brenda grabbed a BVM from the duffel and hooked the device up to the oxygen cylinder. "I'll do compressions," Max said as I took the mask from Brenda.

"You ventilate," she said to me. "I'll hook up the defibrillator."

I pressed the mask of the BVM against the man's face and squeezed the bag, trying to force oxygen into his lungs. Then Max pressed on the man's chest. "One, two. . . ." Suddenly water poured from the man's mouth, filling the mask. "I need suction," I said to Brenda.

She sprinted out the door.

"Oh, yeah," the woman said. "He said he was very thirsty."

I turned the man's face to the side and allowed the water to drain from his mouth and the mask. Then, when Max finished his fifth compression, I again squeezed the bag. More water flowed from the man's mouth and nose. I turned his face but every time Max pressed on the man's chest, more fluid spewed out. "I can't get any air in," I said.

Brenda returned with the suction, and, while I inserted the Yankauer tip into the man's mouth, she turned on the power. Fluid flowed up through the hose and into the suction device's reservoir. "Okay, let's try again."

I refitted the mask and squeezed. More water, and no airway. Again and again we tried to ventilate, using the suction to try to clear his throat, but to no avail.

For ten minutes we continued, frustrated by our inability to create a passage to get oxygen to the man's lungs. My jeans were soaked and I wanted to give up, but once begun, we were committed to continue CPR.

I heard the approaching siren. Amy. Maybe she'd have some idea of how to clear his airway. As we waited for the paramedic, we continued to suction, compress, and try to ventilate. We had already emptied the reservoir of the suction unit twice. How could one man hold so much fluid?

"What's happening?" Amy asked, walking in carrying several canvas bags of equipment.

I told her as much as I had learned. "Older man. Down time before we got here about ten minutes. We've been working."—I glanced at my watch—"about ten minutes more, but I can't get an airway. I don't think we've gotten more than one or two breaths in. He's full of water and every time I try to bag him or Max does a compression, he just belches quarts of the stuff." As if to demonstrate, Max pressed against the man's chest and more water flowed out of his mouth and nose.

Brenda suctioned while Amy hooked up the defibrillator and looked at the EKG screen. "He's flatline." No heart activity at all. "You're unable to ventilate?"

"Totally," I said.

We gazed at the man's face. His lips, cheeks, and jaw were deep blue. Amy took her penlight and shone it into his eyes. The pupils were widely dilated and didn't react at all. She placed her fingers against his throat. "No pulse, and he's getting cold." She lowered her voice. "This is obvious death, especially since you can't ventilate. There's nothing we can do."

I sat back on my haunches and sighed. From outside I heard "Silent Night." Somewhere a clock struck ten.

Sometime later I was working at my computer. More Christmas music was on the radio. I tried to concentrate on my writing, but images of the morning seemed to float on the familiar music.

"O little town of Bethlehem, how still we see thee lie."

After we had stopped CPR a woman had burst into the room, a frantic look on her face. "You can't come in here," I had said to her coldly.

"Above thy deep and dreamless sleep the silent stars go by."

"But I work here. He was my friend," she said, running over to the now-covered, lifeless body on the floor. She bent over and started to remove the sheet from his face, then changed her mind and left it in place. She stood for a moment then turned to me. "I was going to make a party for him," she said. "Tomorrow is his birthday. He always said he was a Christmas present, one day late."

"Yet in thy dark streets shineth the everlasting light."

I wanted to tell her that we had done everything that we could for him. But I looked at her and said nothing. She turned away and left the room.

I sat at my desk, stopped trying to write and let the tears flow. He had only been a "manorite"—one of the strange, disturbed, lost souls who pass time until they die. It had only been a messy code, one that we had been unable to work. He had been only a dead body.

And I was totally unable to deal with the fact that someone cared about him.

"The hopes and fears of all the years are met in thee tonight."

My mother has always been a wonderful and loving parent, supportive, nurturing, and willing to make any sacrifice for my sister or myself. Like many Jewish mothers, however, she also tends to be overprotective, domineering, and impossible to satisfy. She remains so now, even in her nineties. As a child, life with her was a constant, unwinnable struggle.

"Edwin. Eat your soup."

"I'm really not in the mood for soup today, Mom."

"Eat your soup, it's good for you."

"But I don't want any soup today."

"Eat your soup."

I ate the soup. It was easier than arguing. Later, when I hadn't finished the mounds of food that she had placed in front of me, she asked me why I hadn't cleaned my plate. "I just wasn't that hungry, Mom."

"You shouldn't have eaten all that soup. It spoiled your appetite."

Things didn't improve much when I grew up. Last year, as every year, the senior residence in which my mother lives had a New Year's Eve party.

"Come to the party," my mother said.

"I'd love to, Mom," I said, "but I'm scheduled to be on ambulance duty New Year's Eve."

"Come to the party. You'll enjoy it. And you'll be lonely with Joan away."

"Mom, you know how I hate New Year's Eve parties. I'd much rather go to bed early and ignore the holiday completely, unless I get a call. Besides, half the drivers on the road have been drinking and I hate driving on New Year's Eve."

"Come to the party. You'll really enjoy it. There'll be music and dancing and food."

"Mom, you go and have a good time. I'd rather stay home."

"I'm not going to go by myself. What am I going to do there by myself?"

"Mom, all your neighbors will be there. And the people you play cards with."

"No. I'll just stay home if you don't come."

"Okay, Ma, okay. I'll see if I can get someone to cover my ambulance shift. I'll come to the party."

"Edwin, are you sure you want to come? You know how I worry about you driving on New Year's Eve with all the drunken drivers on the road."

When my first daughter, Davida, was born, twenty-five years ago, my mom offered to stay with us for a week and help us with the new baby. It was a disaster. Nothing that my wife or I did was correct. Things came to a head one evening when I cooked dinner.

"These lamb chops are raw," my mom complained.

"They're not raw, Mom. They're not even pink inside. As a matter of fact they are a little overdone."

"I can't eat raw lamb chops," she explained, picking up her plate and disappearing into the kitchen. A few minutes later, black smoke began to billow out of the kitchen.

After the firefighters left, I drove my mom home. It took days to get the blackened residue off the walls, floor, ceiling, and furniture. When we moved to a new apartment, a year later, the apartment still smelled of burned lamb fat.

Although my mom was very proud when she attended a ceremony in which I received a county lifesaving award, she has never really understood why I would voluntarily be with total strangers who are sick or injured. "You could get sick yourself, being with sick people," she frequently admonished. Fortunately, she had never witnessed my being on an actual rescue call until the accident on the parkway a few years ago.

It was a sunny but cool day in October. The autumn leaves in Fairfax were in full color. Joan and I had just picked my mom up and were on our way to my place, where we were all going to spend the day. Nearby was a farm stand that sold cider and doughnuts. It had become somewhat of a tradition to take my mother there every fall. She never tired of seeing the autumn colors, and she loved the doughnuts and cider.

We were driving northbound on the parkway and had just entered Fairfax when we saw the steam rising from the wreckage of the station wagon and the van that apparently had collided just in front of us. What seemed like an endless number of people were pouring out of the wreckage and staggering over to the side of the road. I pulled my car onto the grass beside the pavement. "Joan, why don't you flare out the road. I'll call it in and start triaging."

Although we didn't yet know how many and how serious the injuries were, our first priority was our own safety and the safety of the accident scene. Joan opened the trunk, found a few road flares, and strode down the road, where she would light them and set them out some distance behind the accident scene to warn northbound traffic. My first priority was to call for help. We had to alert the EMS system of a possible MCI—a multiple casualty incident—which might require several emergency response vehicles and additional personnel. I grabbed my portable radio.

"45–22 to GKL–642 Fairfax Ambulance base."

"FVAC on. Go ahead, 45–22."

"I'm at the scene of an MVA on the parkway, about a mile north of the reservoir bridge. Notify the state troopers and have the fire department respond. I don't think there's a fire but there's a lot of steam coming from one of the vehicles. Unknown number and extent of injuries but, judging from the mechanism and the number of people in the vehicles, we may have an MCI. I suggest that you roll the Fairfax duty rig, tone out for standby crews, and put Prescott and Davenport on standby. 45–24 is with me. We'll triage and advise of injuries."

"10–4, 45–22. 45–01 will be en route to your location momentarily and we'll tone out for standby crews for 45–02 and 45–03."

I turned to my mother, who was in the backseat. "Wait in the car, Mom," I said, opening the door.

"You're going out?" she asked.

"Yes, of course, Mom. I have to take care of the people who may be hurt."

"You can't go out without a sweater. It's too cold out. You'll catch a cold."

"Mom, I don't have time to argue with you." I got out of the car, grabbed my crash kit and oxygen tank from the trunk, and began walking toward the accident victims who were standing, sitting, and lying on the grass. Neither Joan nor I would be able to treat anyone until we completed our triage—determination of how many injuries there were and how serious they were—so that we could communicate our response needs to FVAC and decide on priorities for treatment. A number of other cars had stopped at the accident scene and a young woman trotted over to me. "I'm a medic in the city," she said.

"Great," I said. "I'm an EMT with Fairfax Ambulance. I'm in radio contact with local EMS and they're responding. I'm going to check the vehicles for any entrapment. Would you begin triaging the people who are on the grass?"

"Sure," the paramedic responded, and headed toward the mass of people.

I quickly checked both vehicles and determined that there was no one in either of them. I then headed toward Joan, who had finished flaring out the road and was now working with the paramedic on triaging the accident victims. I joined them and while I was asking one of the victims about her injuries, I felt something fall over my shoulders. I spun around and saw my mother standing behind me. I had left the trunk open and she obviously had found the old blanket I keep there and had thrown it over my shoulders. "You'll catch a cold," she explained.

"Mom, I can't wear a blanket while I'm examining people," I said. "Please, wait in the car."

As usual, my protests were useless. "It's cold out. You'll get sick," she said, trying to replace the blanket over my shoulders.

"Mom, wait in the car," I pleaded, but she followed me from patient to patient, demanding that I wear the blanket.

Joan, the medic, and I quickly determined that we had a total of eleven patients, all of whom were stable. There were no life-threatening injuries, just a number of cuts and bruises and two or three possibly fractured limbs. Six of the people had minor injuries to their head or face or were complaining of neck or back pain. These would all have to be collared and boarded. Since none of the patients was critical, two of them could be transported in each ambulance; we would need at least three ambulances plus more for the "walking wounded." I got on the radio and reported our findings, then Joan, the medic, and I began to treat our patients. As we worked, my mother continued to follow me, insisting that I wear the blanket. Soon the air was filled with the wail of sirens as police and fire vehicles arrived and ambulances from three towns began descending on the accident scene.

The most seriously injured person was a twenty-eight-year-old woman with an apparent fracture of the femur, the upper leg bone. She had been dragged out of the car by her husband and was screaming with pain as she lay on the grass. She would be transported by the first ambulance on the scene, but first her leg had to be immobilized with a traction splint.

Applying a traction splint is one of the most dramatic things that an EMT can do. Its application requires a certain amount of skill, and it is used so infrequently that many EMTs have never applied it to a real patient.

The femur is a large, heavy bone that is surrounded by the strongest muscles in the human body. When the femur is broken, these muscles drive the sharp ends of the bones past each other, into the flesh of the thigh. This, plus the cramping of the large muscles surrounding the femur, causes excruciating pain. The traction splint pulls the bone ends slightly back, so that they are no longer being driven into flesh, and stretches the upper leg muscles, relieving their cramping. The result is that, when traction is applied, a patient who is shrieking with pain instantly experiences almost total relief.

Since Joan and I teach traction splinting regularly, I decided that we would be the ones to apply the device. I would hold the woman's foot and pull on it, applying manual traction, while Joan secured the splint in place and turned the ratchet on the device to increase the traction and maintain it during the transport to the hospital. The most important thing about applying a traction splint is that, once manual traction is started, it must be maintained until the device takes over the pulling. If the person who is holding manual traction lets go, the sharp bone ends will spring back, causing additional damage and severe pain. In some instances it can even be fatal, as the bone ends can sever the large femoral artery, causing the patient to bleed to death internally.

I was about to begin pulling on the woman's foot when the blanket fell over my head and I heard my mother's voice behind me. "I can't stand seeing you running around half naked when it's so cold out."

In a rage, I tore the blanket off my head and shoulders. Looking around, I spotted Fairfax Police Officer Stan Poritsky, who was talking to one of the patients. "Stan," I shouted, "can you come over here?"

Stan came over. "What's up, Ed?" he asked.

"Would you please remove this woman from the scene? She's interfering with the work of emergency responders. I'll press charges later if I have to."

Stan grabbed my mother's arm. "Come with me, ma'am," he said politely but firmly, and led her toward the patrol car.

"Oh, and Stan," I called.

Stan stopped and turned toward me, still holding my mother's arm. "Yeah?" he said.

"Be gentle with her. She's my mother."

I couldn't help chuckling at the expression on Stan's face as I turned back toward the patient.

Joan had adjusted the traction splint and nodded to me that she was ready to apply it. From a squatting position I placed my right hand on top of the woman's foot and my left hand around the back of her ankle. Then, rocking backward on my heels, I pulled on, and simultaneously elevated, her leg. At the first movement of her leg, the woman screamed with pain. Then she yelled, "You're pulling my leg out of its socket."

As Joan slid the device into place under the woman's leg, she said, "But it feels better, doesn't it?"

"Oh. Yeah," the woman replied, a surprised expression on her face. "It doesn't hurt now."

After applying the traction splint, we were able to move the woman to the ambulance with relatively little pain.

Fortunately, my mom holds no grudges, and, after the accident scene was cleared and I retrieved her from the back of Stan's patrol car, we went on to see the autumn leaves and had cider and doughnuts. But first I had to stop at my house to get a sweater.

A Final Word

JEMS, the *Journal of Emergency Medical Services*, is one of the major magazines read by EMS volunteers and professionals. Each issue is filled with information on new techniques, tricks, tips, career news, and zillions of advertisements for the "latest" in anything and everything that might interest an emergency medical worker.

A poem originally appeared in the May 1981 issue and was reprinted in August of 1993. Someone who had read one of our earlier books sent us a copy, and we liked it so much that we requested and got permission to reprint it here. We think that it sums up the emergency medical worker better than we ever could.

Song of the EMT
by Thom Dick, EMT-P

Hear me, America.
I am the EMT.
I see your people as never you see them.

Mighty and small, they are beggars before me.
Their faces all frightened
Beseeching

Bewildered and
Hopeful of help from one
More frightened than any . . .

I see their pitiful nakedness,
Their limbs all twisted, their bodies tattered
Their blood on the asphalt
Their children crying.
They trust me to help them.
They know I will help them.

I see their illnesses too, in big cities.
I feel their fevers
As you dream at midnight in small towns.
They call to me whose hearts are aching,
Whose dreams are shattered.
They touch me with their weariness.

Sometimes they seek me who are simply alone,
Who cannot bear the night.
I am their servant, too.

I find them fallen from tractors in fields.
In stilled cars, they are silent and pale on cold rainy
    nights.
The crunching of glass under black heavy boots
Tell my coming.
I fold them in blankets.
I brush back their hair.
I look into their eyes.

My beacons light up their streets as babies are born.
My siren wails down their boulevards

Past their shiny glass walls
Through their stockyards
And past their quiet farms.
People look up from their work as I pass them,
And time is metered in heartbeats.

I fight the battles to keep them alive.
I cover their eyes when they breathe no more.
My partner is a hero
But no one knows his name.

The August 1993 issue of *JEMS* states that the author of this touching work, Paramedic Thom Dick, had retired from EMS after twenty-three years and that he was planning to move to La Mesa, California. If anyone knows how to contact Mr. Dick, please let us know so we may thank him personally. We can be contacted at:

>   Joan Lloyd and Ed Herman
>   PO Box 255
>   Shrub Oak, NY 10588

or via e-mail at JoanELloyd@aol.com.

The Cast

Fairfax Volunteer Ambulance Corps

Radio Call GKL–642
County prefix 45

Emergency Medical Technicians

Nick Abrams—age thirty-five—works split shifts at the local Mobil station.

Stephanie DiMartino—age twenty-two—works in the local Kmart.

Bob Fiorella—age thirty-six—sells insurance and is able to respond to day calls when he's in the area.

Heather Franks—age twenty-five—works in the lunchroom of George Washington Elementary School and goes to college part time.

Tom Franks—age twenty-six—Heather's husband and a second-grade teacher at John Adams Elementary School in Fairfax.

Dave Hancock—age thirty-two—FVAC's Maintenance Officer—auto mechanic at a local auto-body shop.

Ed Herman—age sixty—publisher and biotechnology

specialist who works from his home. Radio call number 45–22.

Pam Kovacs—first lieutenant—age thirty-nine—works part time for a florist. Radio call number 45–12.

Joan Lloyd—age fifty-five—writer who works at home and responds to day calls. Radio call number 45–24.

Jack McCaffrey—age forty-six—professor at Fairfax Community College.

Sam Middleton—age twenty-eight—city firefighter—rides variable shifts as they fit into his schedule.

Steve Nesbitt—age fifty-two—drives a school bus for the Fairfax school system.

Phil Ortiz—age nineteen—became a first responder in the youth corps then, when he became eighteen, he advanced to the senior squad and became an EMT.

Linda Potemski—age forty—emergency room nurse at Fairfax Hospital and a longtime member of FVAC.

Fred Stevens—age forty-three—electrician with a local construction firm.

Marge Talbot—age thirty-five—CPA with a large accounting firm. Frequently works via computer modem and thus can occasionally respond to day calls.

Jill Tremonte—age twenty-one—dental assistant with the Fairfax Dental Group.

Pete Williamson—age twenty-six—professional paramedic with an EMS service in the city.

Probationary Members

Tim Babbett—age twenty-four—works for a local contractor—an EMT but hasn't yet become a full member of the corps.

Davida Herman—age twenty—member of the youth

group who graduated to the senior corps as a probationary member on her eighteenth birthday.

Dispatcher
 Greg Horvath—age sixty-nine—retired plumber.

Fairfax Police Department

 Radio Call ID GBY–639

Officers
 Merve Berkowitz   car 317
 Eileen Flynn   car 318
 Chuck Harding   car 305
 Will McAndrews   car 312
 Stan Poritsky   car 308
 Detective Irv Greenberg

Dispatcher
 Mark Thomas

Fairfax Fire Department

 Radio Call ID GCC–905

Members
 Chief Paul Bradley

Prescott Volunteer Fire Association Rescue Squad

 Radio Call GVK–861
 County prefix 21

Members

Paramedic Amy Chen—age thirty-eight—professional paramedic who began her EMS career with the Prescott Rescue Squad.

EMT Brenda Frost—age thirty-one—works at the local Ford dealership and, when things are quiet, her boss lets her respond to calls.

EMT Ed Herman

EMT Jack Johnson—age forty-three—electrician who has been a member of the Prescott Fire Department since his sixteenth birthday. He joined the rescue squad soon after.

EMT Les Kravitski—age fifty-two—postal worker whose son Evan is also a member of the rescue squad.

EMT Joan Lloyd

Driver Max Taylor—age sixty-eight—retired automobile assembly plant worker who enjoys driving the rescue and responding to emergencies.

EMT Sally Walsh—age twenty-eight—homemaker with three small children; her husband works at home so she can leave when she is needed.

Paramedic Hugh Washington—age twenty-five—professional paramedic with four years of experience.

Prescott Police Department

Radio Call ID GRQ–325

At Fairfax General Hospital ER

Dr. Frank Margolis—emergency medicine specialist
Rosemary Harper, RN—emergency room head nurse
Patty Stewart, RN—emergency room nurse

At St. Luke's Helicopter Service

Sharon Blackstone—flight nurse
Carrie VanWyk—flight nurse

Glossary

4 x 4s—Flat pieces of gauze measuring four inches by four inches, used to cover a wound beneath a bandage.

ALS (advanced life support)—The crew includes at least one paramedic who can perform the life support functions detailed below. See _paramedic_.

AOB—Alcohol on breath.

ASAP—As soon as possible.

backboard—A wooden board approximately six feet long and three feet wide. It is used both as a body splint to support the patient's body and as a lifting aid. Backboards are also called longboards or long spineboards.

BLS (basic life support)—Crew members can perform only the skills of an emergency medical technician with training in defibrillation (EMT-D), despite their level of training.

BP (blood pressure)—An indication of how strongly the heart is beating. Two numbers are usually given. (See *palp.*) The greater number, or systolic pressure, is the pressure when the heart muscle is contracting. The smaller number, or diastolic pressure, is the pressure when the heart muscle is relaxing. A typical blood pressure might be stated as 120 over 80, meaning 120 systolic and 80 diastolic.

brachial artery—The main artery that supplies blood to the arm. The brachial pulse may be felt midway down the upper arm, if fingers are pressed firmly on the inner side, just below the muscle.

BVM (bag valve mask)—A device that forces air or pure oxygen into a patient's lungs. It can be used during CPR or to assist inadequate respirations.

call the code—In the hospital, the staff will continue to work on a person even when the heart has stopped. At some point, however, if the patient doesn't revive, the decision is made to stop. Having made that difficult decision, the doctor in charge will call the code and time of death will be noted.

CCU—Cardiac care unit.

cervical collar—A hard-plastic, specially shaped bracing device that surrounds a patient's neck to prevent additional cervical (neck area) spinal damage. Also called a C-collar.

CISD—Critical incident stress debriefing.

closed fracture—One in which the skin is not broken.

code 2—An ambulance driven code 2 is driven the same way one would drive a car, obeying all traffic laws.

code 3—An ambulance driven code 3, with lights flashing and siren sounding, can disobey most traffic laws. However, the driver is not absolved of the responsibility to drive in a safe and careful manner.

contusion—Bruise.

COPD—Chronic obstructive pulmonary disease.

CPR (cardiopulmonary resuscitation)—The process of using external means to circulate the blood, fill the lungs with oxygen, or both.

crash kit—A container, often international orange, that contains emergency supplies for an EMT to use when assisting a patient. The crash kit, often called a trauma kit, crash bag, or jump bag, contains such supplies as dressings, bandages, scissors, lights, equipment to take vitals, and gloves. EMTs often carry such a kit in their cars. One of the crash kits carried in the ambulance is sometimes called a megaduffel; it contains oxygen supplies, such as an oxygen cylinder, BVM, oral and nasal airways, and various types of masks, in addition to first-aid equipment.

defibrillator—A machine that can deliver an electrical shock to try to "jump-start" a heart that is in v-fib. (See below.) The defibrillator used by the Fairfax EMTs is semiautomatic. The machine assesses the rhythm and decides whether a shock is indicated. If so, it charges and requests that the EMT-D "press to shock." The manual defibrillator that the paramedics use merely shows rhythms on a screen and on a tape. From that information, the medics decide which combination of shock, medications, and/or CPR is indicated.

diaphoretic—Sweaty.

DOA—Dead on arrival.

EDP—Emotionally disturbed person.

EEG (electroencephalogram)—A tracing that shows the electrical activity in the brain.

EKG (electrocardiogram)—A tracing that indicates the electrical activity within the heart's muscle and nervous system.

EMD (electrical mechanical dissociation)—A condition in which electrical impulses in a heart are unable to stimulate normal contractions.

EMT—Emergency medical technician.

EMT-D—An EMT with added training in defibrillation. (See above.) Most of the EMTs in FVAC are EMT-Ds.

ER—Emergency room.

ETA—Estimated time of arrival.

femoral artery—The major blood vessel that supplies blood to the leg. The femoral pulse may be felt in the crease at the upper leg, midway between the hip and groin.

femur—The thigh bone.

FGH—Fairfax General Hospital, the small community hospital that serves the fictional town of Fairfax. In addition to this hospital, down the parkway there is a county medical facility and trauma center.

FVAC—Abbreviation for the fictional Fairfax Volunteer Ambulance Corps. It is pronounced eff vac.

head blocks—Cubes of spongy material covered in heavy plastic that are placed on either side of a victim's head on a long backboard. Placed tightly against the ears and taped down, these blocks keep a patient from moving his or her head and prevent exacerbation of neck injury.

hemothorax—A condition in which blood enters the chest cavity from an internal injury. This prevents a lung from expanding to draw in air.

hot off-load—When a helicopter is delivering a patient to the trauma center and has another call waiting, the pilot does not stop the engines. Rather, he or she leaves the blades turning while the first patient is off-loaded, so the pilot can take off quickly and respond to the second call.

hypovolemic shock—A potentially life-threatening condition (see *shock* below) resulting from severe blood or plasma loss.

intubation—Inserting a tube into a patient's trachea to maintain an open airway.

IV (intravenous line)—A tube inserted into a vein that allows a paramedic, nurse, or doctor to add fluid or medication directly into a patient's blood stream.

jaws of life—A gasoline- or electrically-powered hydraulic tool with several attachments that is used to pry metal from around an entrapped patient. The jaws, also known as the Hurst Tool, are usually used to disentangle a victim from a wrecked automobile.

KED (Kendrick Extrication Device)—A brand-name product. The KED is a plastic-covered, vertically slatted jacket used to immobilize the head, neck, and spine of an accident victim in order to minimize additional trauma while he or she is being moved.

Kling—A brand of roller gauze. Long strips of sterile gauze, prerolled and packaged, that are used to hold a dressing against a wound. Kling tends to adhere to itself, eliminating the necessity for ties or tape.

KVO—Keep vein open.

LOC—Either level of consciousness or loss of consciousness, depending on the situation.

logroll—To turn the body as a unit, to minimize the possibility of increasing any spinal injury. In order to transfer a patient lying on the ground to a backboard, we logroll him or her.

LZ (landing zone)—A helicopter needs a large open area, free of obstructions and overhead wires, in which to land to pick up a patient.

MAST (military antishock trousers)—Pants with inflatable bladders in each leg and the abdomen that can be pressurized like a BP cuff. Inflation is believed to slow the deterioration of a patient in shock. PASG (pneumatic antishock garment) is another acronym for the same apparatus. Currently the efficacy of this device is being debated.

MCI—Multiple casualty incident.

MVA—Motor vehicle accident.

non-rebreather face mask—An oxygen delivery device that consists of a clear plastic mask and a plastic-bag reservoir. When the patient inhales, the reservoir empties, allowing the patient to breathe 100 percent oxygen. As the patient exhales, the air exits through ports at the side of the mask and the reservoir refills from an external oxygen supply.

normal sinus rhythm—The familiar lub-dub rhythm of the heart. This is the normal rhythm of a functioning heart. (See *v-fib* below.)

occlusive dressing—An airtight covering used to keep any air from entering a wound.

open fracture—One in which the skin is broken.

OR—Operating room.

oral airway—Technically called an oropharyngeal airway. This curved breathing tube is inserted into a patient's airway to hold the tongue away from the back of the throat and facilitate ventilations.

palp—Short for palpation. Obtaining a blood pressure by palp means that instead of using a stethoscope to listen to the patient's pulse at the inside of the elbow, the patient's radial pulse (see below) is felt while the BP cuff is deflated.

palpate—Touch a patient's body with light pressure.

paramedic—A member of the emergency medical services who can provide types of patient care beyond an EMT's training. Paramedic care may include invasive procedures such as starting IVs, administering medications, and intubating.

PCR (prehospital care report)—The report that our state requires us to fill out for every call.

PDAA—Property damage auto accident.

pediatric or pede bag—A crash bag containing supplies and equipment in smaller sizes to treat children and infants. In addition, the bag usually contains toys and distractions for younger patients.

PFA—Psychological first aid.

PIAA—Personal injury auto accident.

pneumothorax—A condition in which air enters the chest cavity, preventing a lung from expanding during normal breathing.

point-tenderness—Pain felt when an area of injury is touched or pressed.

prone—Lying facedown.

pronounce—The process of declaring a patient dead. In most states EMTs may not pronounce, whereas paramedics may.

pulses—Places in the body where an artery runs between a bone and the surface. Pulses can be felt with the fingertips. The radial pulse is found in the wrist, the carotid pulse in the neck, the femoral in the groin, and pedal pulses in various locations in the feet.

Reeves—A stretcher consisting of a three-foot-wide assembly of six-foot-long plastic slats covered with plastic. A patient can be placed on the Reeves and the unit wrapped around the body. It keeps the spine supported while allowing the patient to be up-ended or carried at an angle through narrow hallways, over rough terrain, or down stairs. The Reeves has handles at each of the four corners and at the center of each long side, permitting a heavy patient to be lifted more easily.

RMA (refused medical attention)—A competent adult patient always has the right to refuse to let us care for him or her. It is, of course, our job to try to convince an ill or injured person to let us help, but sometimes all our persuasion fails.

shock—The inability of the circulatory system to provide sufficient oxygenated blood to the vital organs.

SOB—Short of breath.

spider strap—An assembly of eight to ten connected straps used to secure a patient quickly to a longboard for transport.

stairchair—A narrow chair with small wheels on the two rear legs and handles for easy carrying. A conscious patient can be seated in the stairchair, belted in, and carried down a flight of stairs or wheeled across a smooth floor.

stat—Immediately. From the Latin *statim*.

supine—Lying on one's back, faceup.

traction splint—A device especially designed to maintain a constant pull along the length of a leg. It is used to stabilize a fracture of the femur (see above) and may help to relieve the muscle spasms that the fracture causes. Traction splints are of two main types, the Hare traction and the Sagar splint.

triage—The process of prioritizing patients when there are more patients than the medical personnel can care for. Assistance is given to those who can gain the most by care.

turnout gear—Coats, pants, hats, and boots made of heavy water- and fireproof material worn by firefighters. We in FVAC wear bright yellow, heavy, lined, weatherproof rain and snow jackets in bad weather.

v-fib—Short for ventricular fibrillation. During ventricular fibrillation, the heart's electrical impulses are disorganized and do not cause the heart to beat well enough to circulate blood throughout the body. Unless v-fib is converted to a normal rhythm, possibly by using a defibrillator, the patient will die.

vitals—Vital signs. Several measurable vitals indicate the stability of a sick or injured person. The vitals we measure are (1) BP (see above); (2) pulse rate and quality; (3) breathing rate and quality; (4) the appearance, temperature, and moistness of the skin; and (5) the response of the pupils of the eyes to light.

water gel—Heavy gauze impregnated with a water-based bacteriacide. These sterile bandages are placed on a burned area to both cool and protect the injury.

Yankauer catheter—A twelve-inch-long hollow plastic tube designed to attach to the end of a suction device's tubing. The Yankauer tip is rigid and can be inserted into the back of the patient's mouth to suction out blood, vomit, and other material that might interfere with the airway.

Authors' Note

Ed and I hope you've enjoyed riding with the wonderful people of the Fairfax Ambulance Corps and the Prescott Volunteer Fire Department Rescue Squad. As you now understand, it's not all television drama and gore. Often it's the small things that are the most rewarding and the most frustrating.

Many of you have been involved in situations like the ones we've described here. We'd love to hear from you, and your story—disguised, of course—might appear in an upcoming book. Please write to us at:

Joan Lloyd and Ed Herman
PO Box 255
Shrub Oak, NY 10588

or e-mail us at: JoanELloyd@aol.com